FREE Test Taking Tips DVD Offer

To help us better serve you, we have developed a Test Taking Tips DVD that we would like to give you for FREE. **This DVD covers world-class test taking tips that you can use to be even more successful when you are taking your test.**

All that we ask is that you email us your feedback about your study guide. Please let us know what you thought about it – whether that is good, bad or indifferent.

To get your **FREE Test Taking Tips DVD**, email freedvd@studyguideteam.com with "FREE DVD" in the subject line and the following information in the body of the email:

    a. The title of your study guide.

    b. Your product rating on a scale of 1-5, with 5 being the highest rating.

    c. Your feedback about the study guide. What did you think of it?

    d. Your full name and shipping address to send your free DVD.

If you have any questions or concerns, please don't hesitate to contact us at freedvd@studyguideteam.com.

Thanks again!

CSCS Study Guide

Exam Prep & Practice Exam Questions for the NSCA Certified Strength & Conditioning Specialist Test

Test Prep Books Certification Prep Team

Table of Contents

Quick Overview

As you draw closer to taking your exam, effective preparation becomes more and more important. Thankfully, you have this study guide to help you get ready. Use this guide to help keep your studying on track and refer to it often.

This study guide contains several key sections that will help you be successful on your exam. The guide contains tips for what you should do the night before and the day of the test. Also included are test-taking tips. Knowing the right information is not always enough. Many well-prepared test takers struggle with exams. These tips will help equip you to accurately read, assess, and answer test questions.

A large part of the guide is devoted to showing you what content to expect on the exam and to helping you better understand that content. In this guide are practice test questions so that you can see how well you have grasped the content. Then, answer explanations are provided so that you can understand why you missed certain questions.

Don't try to cram the night before you take your exam. This is not a wise strategy for a few reasons. First, your retention of the information will be low. Your time would be better used by reviewing information you already know rather than trying to learn a lot of new information. Second, you will likely become stressed as you try to gain a large amount of knowledge in a short amount of time. Third, you will be depriving yourself of sleep. So be sure to go to bed at a reasonable time the night before. Being well-rested helps you focus and remain calm.

Be sure to eat a substantial breakfast the morning of the exam. If you are taking the exam in the afternoon, be sure to have a good lunch as well. Being hungry is distracting and can make it difficult to focus. You have hopefully spent lots of time preparing for the exam. Don't let an empty stomach get in the way of success!

When travelling to the testing center, leave earlier than needed. That way, you have a buffer in case you experience any delays. This will help you remain calm and will keep you from missing your appointment time at the testing center.

Be sure to pace yourself during the exam. Don't try to rush through the exam. There is no need to risk performing poorly on the exam just so you can leave the testing center early. Allow yourself to use all of the allotted time if needed.

Remain positive while taking the exam even if you feel like you are performing poorly. Thinking about the content you should have mastered will not help you perform better on the exam.

Once the exam is complete, take some time to relax. Even if you feel that you need to take the exam again, you will be well served by some down time before you begin studying again. It's often easier to convince yourself to study if you know that it will come with a reward!

Test-Taking Strategies

1. Predicting the Answer

When you feel confident in your preparation for a multiple-choice test, try predicting the answer before reading the answer choices. This is especially useful on questions that test objective factual knowledge. By predicting the answer before reading the available choices, you eliminate the possibility that you will be distracted or led astray by an incorrect answer choice. You will feel more confident in your selection if you read the question, predict the answer, and then find your prediction among the answer choices. After using this strategy, be sure to still read all of the answer choices carefully and completely. If you feel unprepared, you should not attempt to predict the answers. This would be a waste of time and an opportunity for your mind to wander in the wrong direction.

2. Reading the Whole Question

Too often, test takers scan a multiple-choice question, recognize a few familiar words, and immediately jump to the answer choices. Test authors are aware of this common impatience, and they will sometimes prey upon it. For instance, a test author might subtly turn the question into a negative, or he or she might redirect the focus of the question right at the end. The only way to avoid falling into these traps is to read the entirety of the question carefully before reading the answer choices.

3. Looking for Wrong Answers

Long and complicated multiple-choice questions can be intimidating. One way to simplify a difficult multiple-choice question is to eliminate all of the answer choices that are clearly wrong. In most sets of answers, there will be at least one selection that can be dismissed right away. If the test is administered on paper, the test taker could draw a line through it to indicate that it may be ignored; otherwise, the test taker will have to perform this operation mentally or on scratch paper. In either case, once the obviously incorrect answers have been eliminated, the remaining choices may be considered. Sometimes identifying the clearly wrong answers will give the test taker some information about the correct answer. For instance, if one of the remaining answer choices is a direct opposite of one of the eliminated answer choices, it may well be the correct answer. The opposite of obviously wrong is obviously right! Of course, this is not always the case. Some answers are obviously incorrect simply because they are irrelevant to the question being asked. Still, identifying and eliminating some incorrect answer choices is a good way to simplify a multiple-choice question.

4. Don't Overanalyze

Anxious test takers often overanalyze questions. When you are nervous, your brain will often run wild, causing you to make associations and discover clues that don't actually exist. If you feel that this may be a problem for you, do whatever you can to slow down during the test. Try taking a deep breath or counting to ten. As you read and consider the question, restrict yourself to the particular words used by the author. Avoid thought tangents about what the author *really* meant, or what he or she was *trying* to say. The only things that matter on a multiple-choice test are the words that are actually in the question. You must avoid reading too much into a multiple-choice question, or supposing that the writer meant something other than what he or she wrote.

5. No Need for Panic

It is wise to learn as many strategies as possible before taking a multiple-choice test, but it is likely that you will come across a few questions for which you simply don't know the answer. In this situation, avoid panicking. Because most multiple-choice tests include dozens of questions, the relative value of a single wrong answer is small. As much as possible, you should compartmentalize each question on a multiple-choice test. In other words, you should not allow your feelings about one question to affect your success on the others. When you find a question that you either don't understand or don't know how to answer, just take a deep breath and do your best. Read the entire question slowly and carefully. Try rephrasing the question a couple of different ways. Then, read all of the answer choices carefully. After eliminating obviously wrong answers, make a selection and move on to the next question.

6. Confusing Answer Choices

When working on a difficult multiple-choice question, there may be a tendency to focus on the answer choices that are the easiest to understand. Many people, whether consciously or not, gravitate to the answer choices that require the least concentration, knowledge, and memory. This is a mistake. When you come across an answer choice that is confusing, you should give it extra attention. A question might be confusing because you do not know the subject matter to which it refers. If this is the case, don't eliminate the answer before you have affirmatively settled on another. When you come across an answer choice of this type, set it aside as you look at the remaining choices. If you can confidently assert that one of the other choices is correct, you can leave the confusing answer aside. Otherwise, you will need to take a moment to try to better understand the confusing answer choice. Rephrasing is one way to tease out the sense of a confusing answer choice.

7. Your First Instinct

Many people struggle with multiple-choice tests because they overthink the questions. If you have studied sufficiently for the test, you should be prepared to trust your first instinct once you have carefully and completely read the question and all of the answer choices. There is a great deal of research suggesting that the mind can come to the correct conclusion very quickly once it has obtained all of the relevant information. At times, it may seem to you as if your intuition is working faster even than your reasoning mind. This may in fact be true. The knowledge you obtain while studying may be retrieved from your subconscious before you have a chance to work out the associations that support it. Verify your instinct by working out the reasons that it should be trusted.

8. Key Words

Many test takers struggle with multiple-choice questions because they have poor reading comprehension skills. Quickly reading and understanding a multiple-choice question requires a mixture of skill and experience. To help with this, try jotting down a few key words and phrases on a piece of scrap paper. Doing this concentrates the process of reading and forces the mind to weigh the relative importance of the question's parts. In selecting words and phrases to write down, the test taker thinks about the question more deeply and carefully. This is especially true for multiple-choice questions that are preceded by a long prompt.

9. Subtle Negatives

One of the oldest tricks in the multiple-choice test writer's book is to subtly reverse the meaning of a question with a word like *not* or *except*. If you are not paying attention to each word in the question, you can easily be led astray by this trick. For instance, a common question format is, "Which of the following is...?" Obviously, if the question instead is, "Which of the following is not...?," then the answer will be quite different. Even worse, the test makers are aware of the potential for this mistake and will include one answer choice that would be correct if the question were not negated or reversed. A test taker who misses the reversal will find what he or she believes to be a correct answer and will be so confident that he or she will fail to reread the question and discover the original error. The only way to avoid this is to practice a wide variety of multiple-choice questions and to pay close attention to each and every word.

10. Reading Every Answer Choice

It may seem obvious, but you should always read every one of the answer choices! Too many test takers fall into the habit of scanning the question and assuming that they understand the question because they recognize a few key words. From there, they pick the first answer choice that answers the question they believe they have read. Test takers who read all of the answer choices might discover that one of the latter answer choices is actually *more* correct. Moreover, reading all of the answer choices can remind you of facts related to the question that can help you arrive at the correct answer. Sometimes, a misstatement or incorrect detail in one of the latter answer choices will trigger your memory of the subject and will enable you to find the right answer. Failing to read all of the answer choices is like not reading all of the items on a restaurant menu: you might miss out on the perfect choice.

11. Spot the Hedges

One of the keys to success on multiple-choice tests is paying close attention to every word. This is never truer than with words like almost, most, some, and sometimes. These words are called "hedges" because they indicate that a statement is not totally true or not true in every place and time. An absolute statement will contain no hedges, but in many subjects, the answers are not always straightforward or absolute. There are always exceptions to the rules in these subjects. For this reason, you should favor those multiple-choice questions that contain hedging language. The presence of qualifying words indicates that the author is taking special care with his or her words, which is certainly important when composing the right answer. After all, there are many ways to be wrong, but there is only one way to be right! For this reason, it is wise to avoid answers that are absolute when taking a multiple-choice test. An absolute answer is one that says things are either all one way or all another. They often include words like *every*, *always*, *best*, and *never*. If you are taking a multiple-choice test in a subject that doesn't lend itself to absolute answers, be on your guard if you see any of these words.

12. Long Answers

In many subject areas, the answers are not simple. As already mentioned, the right answer often requires hedges. Another common feature of the answers to a complex or subjective question are qualifying clauses, which are groups of words that subtly modify the meaning of the sentence. If the question or answer choice describes a rule to which there are exceptions or the subject matter is complicated, ambiguous, or confusing, the correct answer will require many words in order to be expressed clearly and accurately. In essence, you should not be deterred by answer choices that seem excessively long. Oftentimes, the author of the text will not be able to write the correct answer without offering some qualifications and modifications. Your job is to read the answer choices thoroughly and completely and to select the one that most accurately and precisely answers the question.

13. Restating to Understand

Sometimes, a question on a multiple-choice test is difficult not because of what it asks but because of how it is written. If this is the case, restate the question or answer choice in different words. This process serves a couple of important purposes. First, it forces you to concentrate on the core of the question. In order to rephrase the question accurately, you have to understand it well. Rephrasing the question will concentrate your mind on the key words and ideas. Second, it will present the information to your mind in a fresh way. This process may trigger your memory and render some useful scrap of information picked up while studying.

14. True Statements

Sometimes an answer choice will be true in itself, but it does not answer the question. This is one of the main reasons why it is essential to read the question carefully and completely before proceeding to the answer choices. Too often, test takers skip ahead to the answer choices and look for true statements. Having found one of these, they are content to select it without reference to the question above. Obviously, this provides an easy way for test makers to play tricks. The savvy test taker will always read the entire question before turning to the answer choices. Then, having settled on a correct answer choice, he or she will refer to the original question and ensure that the selected answer is relevant. The mistake of choosing a correct-but-irrelevant answer choice is especially common on questions related to specific pieces of objective knowledge. A prepared test taker will have a wealth of factual knowledge at his or her disposal, and should not be careless in its application.

15. No Patterns

One of the more dangerous ideas that circulates about multiple-choice tests is that the correct answers tend to fall into patterns. These erroneous ideas range from a belief that B and C are the most common right answers, to the idea that an unprepared test-taker should answer "A-B-A-C-A-D-A-B-A." It cannot be emphasized enough that pattern-seeking of this type is exactly the WRONG way to approach a multiple-choice test. To begin with, it is highly unlikely that the test maker will plot the correct answers according to some predetermined pattern. The questions are scrambled and delivered in a random order. Furthermore, even if the test maker was following a pattern in the assignation of correct answers, there is no reason why the test taker would know which pattern he or she was using. Any attempt to discern a pattern in the answer choices is a waste of time and a distraction from the real work of taking the test. A test taker would be much better served by extra preparation before the test than by reliance on a pattern in the answers.

FREE DVD OFFER

Don't forget that doing well on your exam includes both understanding the test content and understanding how to use what you know to do well on the test. We offer a completely FREE Test Taking Tips DVD that covers world class test taking tips that you can use to be even more successful when you are taking your test.

All that we ask is that you email us your feedback about your study guide. To get your **FREE Test Taking Tips DVD**, email freedvd@studyguideteam.com with "FREE DVD" in the subject line and the following information in the body of the email:

- The title of your study guide.
- Your product rating on a scale of 1-5, with 5 being the highest rating.
- Your feedback about the study guide. What did you think of it?
- Your full name and shipping address to send your free DVD.

Introduction to the CSCS Exam

Function of the Test

The CSCS exam is a two-part test required to receive qualification as a Certified Strength and Conditioning Specialist (CSCS). The role of CSCS experts is to help improve the physical performance of athletes of all ages and abilities, from beginner to professional, while minimizing the risk of injury. The exam measures candidates' aptitude regarding the scientific foundations and practical applications of strength training and conditioning. Exams are held in test centers around the world.

CSCS exam candidates residing in the U.S. must have a bachelor's degree or be current registered college seniors at an accredited school. In addition, candidates must have Cardiopulmonary Resuscitation (CPR) and Automated External Defibrillator (AED) certification cards from an accepted association, such as the American Heart Association or the Red Cross. Those living outside the United States and Canada must have a bachelor's degree recognized by U.S. educational standards, or confirm enrollment as a college senior at an institution acknowledged by that nation as a degree-granting college or university.

Candidates typically have educational or professional experience in one of the following specialties: exercise science/physiology, strength training and conditioning, kinesiology and biomechanics, or physical therapy and athletic training. According to the National Strength and Conditioning Association (NSCA), the organization that develops and administers the examination, 3,589 examinees took both sections of the CSCS test between July 2012 and June 2013. The current pass rate for the CSCS exam is 63%.

Test Administration

CSCS exams are offered throughout the year at Pearson VUE test locations worldwide. There are separate fees for NSCA members and non-members. Full-time college students can obtain a NSCA student membership; alternatively, professional memberships are also available. First-time test takers need to register and take both sections (Scientific Foundations and Practical/Applied). Examinees who achieve a passing grade on both test sections receive CSCS accreditation. However, if a candidate receives a passing score on just one section, he or she may retake the failed section and thus obtain certification upon receipt of a passing grade. There are applicable fees to retake the entire exam or just one section.

Although there are no restrictions on the number of times a candidate may retake the CSCS exam, he or she must wait 90 days to retest. Eligibility requirements do not need to be resubmitted unless prior CPR/AED certification has expired. Pearson VUE will honor special test arrangements for examinees with disabilities upon request.

Test Format

There are two parts of the CSCS exam: Scientific Foundations and Practical/Applied.

The Scientific Foundations section has a total of 95 multiple-choice questions – 80 that are scored and 15 that are not scored. The Practical/Applied exam incudes 125 multiple-choice questions – 110 that scored and 15 that are not scored. The total time to take both sections is about four hours. There is a break between the two parts that is not included in this time estimation.

The non-scored questions are distributed throughout the exam so that individuals will give them the same amount of attention as the scored questions. Under evaluation by the CSCS Exam Development Committee for potential future use, these pretest questions may be included on forthcoming CSCS exams as scored questions. These non-scored questions are not included in a candidate's official score and do not impact pass/fail status.

The Scientific Foundations section of the CSCS exam is meant to measure a candidate's exercise science skills, specifically in areas such as anatomy, exercise physiology, biomechanics, and nutrition. The length of time to take this section is one and a half hours.

Scientific Foundations Section

Total time = 1.5 hours

Field	Percent of Section	Number of Questions
Exercise Science	74%	59
Nutrition	26%	21
Non-scored Questions		15
Total	**100%**	**95**

The Practical/Applied section is two and a half hours and focuses on program design, exercise techniques, testing and evaluation, and organization and administration. This section includes 30-40 electronic and/or visual prompts that measure knowledge in the areas of exercise techniques, functional anatomy, and testing procedures.

Practical/Applied Section

Total Time = 2.5 hours

Field	Percent of Section	Number of Questions
Exercise Technique	35%	38
Program Design	35%	39
Organization and Administration	12%	13
Testing and Evaluation	18%	20
Non-scored Questions		15
Total	**100%**	**125**

Scoring

Each part of the CSCS exam is graded on a point scale of 1 to 99, with 70 considered a passing score. Scaled scores can be compared across the various exam formulations, which may have somewhat different levels of complexity. For example, a scaled score of 75 received in 2014 is equal to a scaled score of 75 received in 2016, even though the two exams may have contained slightly different questions. Statistical techniques to equalize the CSCS exams are used to make sure the different exam formulations maintain the same standard of difficulty. A candidate's strong and weak points are depicted as raw (unscaled) domain scores. Raw scores cannot be directly associated to scaled scores.

Exercise Sciences

Muscle Anatomy

Muscle Groups by Region

There are over 500 skeletal muscles in the body, so muscles are often grouped together in various ways to simplify learning and to enhance application of muscular knowledge for practical purposes. For resistance training programs, muscles are often grouped by body region or movement. By considering muscles by groups, it is easier to develop a targeted resistance training program or implement split routine workouts. For example, thirteen muscle groups associated with individual body regions can be broken into two or three training groups that are rotated during a week of training.

Upper body: biceps (front of upper arms), rectus and transverse abdominus (stomach), deltoids (top of shoulders), latissimus dorsi and rhomboids (back and between shoulder blades), pectoralis major and minor (front of upper chest), obliques (side of torso), trapezius (upper/mid back), triceps (back of upper arms), etc.

Lower body: quadriceps (front of thighs), erector spinae (lower back), gastrocnemius and soleus (back of lower legs), gluteus major and minor (buttocks), hamstrings (back of thighs), adductors (inner thigh), etc.

Muscle Groups by Function

Muscles are also frequently grouped according to the movements they help produce or control. This is often called functional anatomy and is particularly important when assessing an athlete's movement dysfunction, imbalance, or injury pattern. The typical functional groups include muscles for 1) facial expression, 2) mastication, 3) head and vertebral column movement, 4) pectoral girdle movement, 5) arm movement, 6) forearm movement, 7) hand movement, 8) abdominal wall movement, 9) pelvic outlet movement, 10) thigh movement, 11) leg movement, and 12) foot movement.

Muscles Involved in Arm, Forearm, and Hand Movement

There are four primary actions associated with arm movement. Arm (humerus) or shoulder flexion is carried out by pectoralis major, the anterior fibers of the deltoid, and coracobrachialis. Teres major, latissimus dorsi, and the posterior fibers of the deltoid are the muscles are responsible for arm or shoulder extension. The supraspinatus and deltoid muscles are responsible for arm abduction, and the subscapularis, infraspinatus, and teres minor muscles rotate the arm.

The biceps brachii, brachialis, and brachioradialis muscles are responsible for elbow flexion, which lifts the forearm. The triceps brachii and the anconeus control elbow and forearm extension. The supinator, pronator teres, and pronator quadratus muscles rotate the forearm.

Compared to the arm and forearm, a greater number of muscles are responsible for the flexion and extension of the wrist, hand, and fingers. Flexion of the wrist and hand results from the actions of the flexor carpi radialis, flexor carpi ulnaris, palmaris longus, flexor digitorum profundus, and flexor digitorum superficialis muscles. There are even smaller muscles that control thumb and digit flexion. Wrist and hand extension results from the movements of the extensor carpi radialis longus, extensor carpi radialis brevis, extensor carpi ulnaris, and extensor digitorum muscles. In general, large gross movements are usually produced by fewer, but stronger muscles, while fine, coordinated movements involve many small muscles working in concert with one another to execute precise actions.

Muscles Involved in Leg and Foot Movement

Knee flexion results from the hamstring group of muscles (biceps femoris, semitendinosus, semimembranosus) and the sartorius muscle. Knee extension is carried out by the quadriceps femoris group of muscles (rectus femoris, vastus lateralis, vastus medialis, and vastus intermedius).

Dorsiflexion (lifting the foot up) of the ankle results from the movement of the tibialis anterior, fibularis tertius, extensor digitorum longus, and extensor hallucis longus muscles. The gastrocnemius, soleus, plantaris, and flexor digitorum longus are responsible for ankle plantarflexion. Inversion (medial movement) and eversion (lateral movement) of the foot are controlled by the tibialis posterior and fibularis longus muscles, respectively.

Orientation/Directional/Regional Anatomical Terms

The following anatomical terms are commonly used in the description of muscle origins, insertions, and actions:

Superior (cranial): Near or toward the upper part of the body, i.e., toward the head. The clavicle is superior to the iliac crest.

Inferior (caudal): Toward the lower part of a structure or the body and away from the head. The talus is inferior to the patella.

Anterior (ventral): At or near the front of the body. The sternum is anterior to the spine.

Posterior (dorsal): At or near the back of the body. The spine is posterior to the sternum.

Medial: Near or at the body's midline. The nose is medial to the ears.

Lateral: Away from the body's midline. The ears are lateral to the nose.

Bilateral: On either side of a central axis or midline. The body has many bilateral (paired) structures including the legs, eyes, lungs, etc.

Ipsilateral: On or affecting the same side of the body. Ipsilateral appendages (e.g., hands and feet) are located on the same side of the body.

Contralateral: On or affecting the opposite sides of the body. A stroke that occurs on the right side of the brain may affect the function of the left arm.

Intermediate: Located between two structures—one that is medial and one that is lateral or one that is superior and one that is inferior. The knee is intermediate to the ankle and hip.

Proximal: Location of the origin or point of attachment of the body part towards the trunk and away from the appendages. The thigh is proximal to the ankle.

Distal: Location of the origin or point of attachment being away from the body. The ankle is distal to the knee.

Superficial (external): Near the outside or surface of an object or body.

Deep (internal): Inside, away from the surface of an object or body.

Axial: Associated with the center of the body. When considering the skeleton, the body's head, neck, and trunk make up the axial skeleton.

Appendicular: Refers to the body's appendages, such as the legs and arms.

Abduct: A movement away from the body's midline. When doing jumping jacks, the first phase of the arm movement abducts away from the side of the body en route to its position above the head.

Adduct: A movement toward the body's midline. The second phase of the arm movement during jumping jacks (returning them back in line with the trunk) demonstrates adduction.

Specific Muscle Names

One of the easiest ways to remember specific muscle names is to group the muscles by body regions. The following table of muscles, grouped by region, provides the name and action of the muscle as well as the origin (the anchoring end of the skeletal muscle, typically on a bone) and insertion (the end of the skeletal muscle that attaches to the bone or tissue that moves during the contraction). Muscles that are of primary relevance (e.g., muscles critical for sport/activity movements and muscles that aid respiration) to the strength and conditioning professional are included in this list. Examples of resistance exercises that target specific muscles are also provided. Please bear in mind that this is not an exhaustive list, but rather covers the most relevant muscles for coaches.

Muscle	Origin (immovable end of muscle)	Insertion (movable end of muscle)	Action	Resistance Exercise(s)
Erector spinae: iliocostalis (most lateral), longissimus (intermediate), spinalis (most medial)	Varies for each column	Varies for each column	Prime mover of back extension; each side consists of three columns (iliocostalis, longissimus, and spinalis muscles).	Seated rows Dumbbell rows Power jerk Stiff-leg dead lift Dead lifts Back extensions Lumbar extensions
Trapezius	Occipital bone, ligamentum nuchae, and spines of C7 and all thoracic vertebrae	A continuous insertion along acromion and spine of scapula and lateral third of clavicle	Stabilizes, raises, and rotates scapula; middle fibers retract (adduct) scapula; superior fibers elevate scapula (i.e., shrugging shoulders); inferior fibers depress scapula (and shoulder).	Back presses Bent-over lateral raises Arnold presses Lateral dumbbell raises Chin-ups Seated cable rows Dumbbell rows Dead lifts Power clean Power snatch Power jerk Lateral pull-downs Machine shoulder press Dumbbell prone posterior raise

Muscle	Origin (immovable end of muscle)	Insertion (movable end of muscle)	Action	Resistance Exercise(s)
Rhomboid major	Spinous processes of T2-T5	Medial (i.e., vertebral) border of scapula	Retracts, elevates, and rotates scapula	Dead lift Bent-over lateral raises Alternate front arm raises Dumbbell pull-overs Chin-ups Dumbbell one-arm row Seated cable rows Lateral pull-downs
Rhomboid minor	Spinous processes of C7-T1	Medial border of scapula	Retracts and elevates scapula	Dead lift Bent-over lateral raises Alternate front arm raises Dumbbell pull-overs Chin-ups Dumbbell one-arm row Lateral pull-downs Seated cable rows
Levator scapulae	Transverse processes of C1-C4	Medial border of scapula	Elevates scapula; flexes neck to same side	Dead lifts
Serratus anterior	Series of muscle slips from ribs	Entire anterior (ventral) surface of vertebral border of scapula	Pulls scapula anteriorly and downward; abducts scapula	Back presses Arnold presses Alternate front arm raises Incline dumbbell press Dumbbell pull-overs Bench press, dumbbell Dumbbell fly Machine shoulder press

Muscle	Origin (immovable end of muscle)	Insertion (movable end of muscle)	Action	Resistance Exercise(s)
Pectoralis minor	Anterior surfaces of ribs three through five	Coracoid process of scapula	Abducts scapula, pulling it forward and downward; draws rib cage superiorly (raises ribs)	Incline dumbbell press Dumbbell pull-overs Bench press, dumbbell Bench press, barbell Incline press, dumbbell Dumbbell fly
Pectoralis major	Medial 1/2 of clavicle, sternum, and costal cartilages of ribs one through six	Greater tubercle of humerus	Prime mover of arm flexion; rotates arm medially, adducts humerus; pulls arm across chest	Triceps dips Arnold presses Alternate front arm raises Push-ups Barbell pull-overs Bench press, dumbbell Dumbbell fly
Teres major	Posterior surface of scapula at inferior angle	Intertubercular groove of humerus	Posteromedially extends, medially rotates, and adducts humerus; synergist of latissimus dorsi	Dumbbell pull-overs Barbell pull-overs Chin-ups Lateral pull-downs Dead lifts Dumbbell one-arm row Lateral pull-downs Seated cable rows
Latissimus dorsi	Spines of lower six thoracic vertebrae, lumbar vertebrae, lower three to four ribs, and iliac crest	Intertubercular groove of humerus	Prime mover of arm extension; arm adductor; medially rotates humerus at shoulder	Dumbbell pull-overs Barbell pull-overs Chin-ups Lateral pull-downs Seated rows Dead lifts Dumbbell one-arm row Seated cable rows

Muscle	Origin (immovable end of muscle)	Insertion (movable end of muscle)	Action	Resistance Exercise(s)
Deltoids	Spine of scapula, acromion, and lateral 1/3 of clavicle	Deltoid tuberosity of humerus	Prime mover of arm abduction (at shoulder); extends and flexes arm	Dead lift Triceps dips (anterior deltoid) Back presses Bent-over lateral raises Lateral dumbbell raises Alternate front arm raises Push-ups Seated cable rows Dumbbell rows Power clean Power snatch Power jerk Bench press, dumbbell Dumbbell fly Dumbbell one-arm row Lateral pull-downs Machine shoulder press Dumbbell prone posterior raise
Rotator cuff: supraspinatus, infraspinatus, teres minor, subscapularis	Varies for each muscle	Varies for each muscle	Medially or laterally rotates arm at shoulder; supraspinatus assists abduction; stabilizes shoulder joint, helping to prevent downward dislocation of humerus	Back presses Bent-over lateral raises Dumbbell rows Dumbbell prone posterior raise
Biceps brachii	Short head: coracoid process of scapula; long head: tubercle above glenoid cavity of scapula	Radial tuberosity of radius	Flexes elbow joint and supinates forearm and hand	Dumbbell curl Hammer curl Barbell curls Chin-ups Lateral pull-downs Dumbbell one-arm row Seated cable rows

Muscle	Origin (immovable end of muscle)	Insertion (movable end of muscle)	Action	Resistance Exercise(s)
Brachialis	Anterior, distal 1/2 of humerus	Coronoid process of ulna	Flexes elbow	Dumbbell curl Hammer curls Barbell curls Chin-ups Lateral pull-downs Dumbbell one-arm row Seated cable rows
Brachioradialis	Lateral supracondylar ridge at distal end of humerus	Base of styloid process of radius	Flexes forearm at elbow	Hammer curls Dumbbell curls Barbell curls Chin-ups Seated rows Dumbbell one-arm row Lateral pull-downs Seated cable rows
Triceps brachii	Long head: infraglenoid tubercle of scapula; lateral head: posterior humerus above radial groove; medial head: posterior humerus below	All three heads: olecranon process of ulna	Extends forearm at elbow	Push-downs Reverse push-downs Lying dumbbell triceps extensions Triceps kickbacks Seated dumbbell triceps extensions Triceps dips Back presses Arnold presses Push-ups Dumbbell pull-overs Power snatch Bench press, dumbbell Machine shoulder press
External oblique	Outer surfaces of lower eight ribs	Outer lip of iliac crest and linea alba	Tenses abdominal wall and compresses abdominal contents	Dead lifts Sit-ups Leg raises Dumbbell side bends Abdominal crunch
Internal oblique	Lumbar fascia, iliac crest, and inguinal ligament	Cartilages of lower ribs, linea alba, and crest of pubis	Tenses abdominal wall and compresses abdominal contents	Dumbbell side bends

Muscle	Origin (immovable end of muscle)	Insertion (movable end of muscle)	Action	Resistance Exercise(s)
Transverse abdominis	Inguinal ligament, lumbar fascia, cartilages of last six ribs, iliac crest	Linea alba and crest of pubis	Compresses abdominal components	Pelvic floor exercises Planks
Rectus abdominis	Crest of pubis and symphysis pubis	Xiphoid process and costal cartilages of ribs five through seven	Flexes and rotates lumbar region of vertebral column; fixes and depresses ribs, stabilizes pelvis when walking; tenses abdominal wall, increases intra-abdominal pressure	Dead lifts Sit-ups Leg raises Dumbbell side bends Abdominal crunch
Psoas major (iliopsoas)	Lumbar intervertebral discs; bodies and transverse processes of lumbar vertebrae	Lesser trochanter of femur via iliopsoas tendon	Flexes thigh; also affects lateral flexion of vertebral column; important postural muscle	Leg raises Barbell lunge
Iliacus (iliopsoas)	Iliac fossa and crest, lateral sacrum	Femur on and immediately below lesser trochanter of femur via iliopsoas tendon	Prime mover for flexing thigh or for flexing trunk on thigh during a bow	Leg raises Barbell lunge
Gluteus maximus	Sacrum, coccyx, and posterior surface of ilium	Posterior surface of femur and fascia of thigh	Major extensor of thigh; generally inactive during standing and walking; laterally rotates and abducts thigh	Dead lifts Power clean Power snatch Power jerk Back squat Front squat Barbell lunge Stiff-leg dead lift Leg press Back extensions
Piriformis	Anterior surface of sacrum	Superior border of greater trochanter of femur	Abducts and rotates thigh laterally; stabilizes hip joint	Dead lifts

Muscle	Origin (immovable end of muscle)	Insertion (movable end of muscle)	Action	Resistance Exercise(s)
Hamstring group: biceps femoris, semitendinosus, semimembranosus	Ischial tuberosity (specifics vary on muscle)	Varies on muscle	Extends thigh and flexes knee; laterally or medially rotates leg, especially when knee is flexed	Dead lifts Standing leg curls Seated leg curls Power clean Power snatch Power jerk Back squat Front squat Barbell lunge Stiff-leg dead lift Leg press Leg curl Back extensions
Quadriceps group: vastus lateralis, medialis and intermedius, rectus femoris	Varies on specific muscle	Patellar ligament to tibial tuberosity	Extends and stabilizes knee	Dead lifts Leg extensions Power clean Power snatch Power jerk Back squat Front squat Barbell lunge Leg press
Gastrocnemius	Lateral and medial condyles of femur	Posterior surface of calcaneus	Plantar flexion of foot; flexes knee	Standing leg curls Seated leg curls Standing calf raises Power clean Power snatch Power jerk Barbell lunge Standing heel raise
Soleus	Head and shaft of fibula and posterior surface of tibia	Posterior surface of calcaneus	Plantar flexion of foot	Standing calf raises Power clean Power snatch Power jerk Barbell lunge

Muscle Belly Anatomy

Muscle fibers: Also called muscle cells or myocytes, muscle fibers are long, striated, cylindrical cells approximately the diameter of a human hair (50-100 micrometers). Many nuclei are dispersed throughout the cell, which is covered by a fibrous membrane called the sarcolemma. Up to 150 muscle fibers can be bundled together into parallel fasciculi, with each fasciculus covered by perimysium (i.e., connective tissue) and each muscle fiber covered by endomysium, another type of connective tissue.

Sarcolemma: A thin elastic membrane consisting of a phospholipid bilayer (like eukaryotic cell membranes) and an outer membrane with collagen and other structural elements, which surrounds each muscle fiber.

Sarcoplasm: Sarcoplasm is the special term for the cytoplasm of a muscle fiber. Sarcoplasm is filled with myofibrils and contains the components required for muscular contraction, including various proteins, protein filaments, mitochondria, the sarcoplasmic reticulum, stored glycogen, enzymes, and ions.

Sarcoplasmic reticulum: The sarcoplasmic reticulum is a network of tubular channels (i.e., transverse [T]-tubule system) and vesicles, which together provide structural integrity to the muscle fiber. The sarcoplasmic reticulum also acts as a calcium ion (Ca^{2+}) pump, moving Ca^{2+} ions from the sarcoplasm into the muscle fiber. Influx of Ca^{2+} ions from the sarcoplasm into the muscle fiber results from an action potential in the sarcomere, causing the depolarization that initiates muscle movement.

Myofibril: Myofibrils consist of long, thin (approximately 1/1000 millimeter) chain proteins, such as actin, myosin, and titan. Bunches of myofibrils and nuclei together make a muscle fiber.

Myofilament: Myofilaments primarily consist of protein chains containing actin and myosin and are the smaller components of the myofibrils within striated muscle fibers. A sarcomere is composed of myofilaments.

Sarcomere: The smallest functional unit of a muscle fiber, a sarcomere contains the actin and myosin proteins responsible for the mechanical process of muscle contractions. Located between two Z-lines, actin and myosin filaments are configured in parallel, end to end, along the entire length of the myofibril. The varying arrangement of actin and myosin segments within the sarcomere causes the alternating light and dark pattern of skeletal muscle seen histologically. The sarcomere has four defined segments: A-band, H-zone, I-band, and Z-line. Each sarcomere is composed of a basic repeating unit between the Z-line located at each end of the sarcomere. The A-band contains both actin and myosin. The H-zone, a region located in the center of the sarcomere within the A-band, contains only myosin filaments. The I-band contains only actin filaments and consists of two connected sarcomeres on either side of the Z-line.

Transverse tubular system: The T-tubular system is perpendicular to the myofibril and two sarcoplasmic channels. The lateral end of each tubule channel terminates as a Ca^2 storing vesicle. Each Z-line region contains two vesicles and a T-tubule. T-tubules pass through the muscle cell, open externally from the inside of the cell, and touch the sarcolemma on the surface of the cell. The vesicles and T-tubules spread the action potential (i.e., wave of depolarization) from the surface of the cell's outer membrane to all inner regions of the cell. Depolarization releases Ca^{2+} from vesicles, initiating contractile motion.

Myosin: The interaction between myosin, the thick filament, and actin, the thin filament, causes the sarcomere to shorten as the muscle contracts. Myosin is often described as resembling a bunch of golf clubs, with the heads forming the attachment site along the actin myofilaments, which resemble a string of beads. Myosin is also responsible for splitting adenosine triphosphate (ATP). The phosphate released from ATP hydrolysis provides the energy required for myosin to produce the power stroke, causing the myosin head to grab onto the actin and pull the filaments closer together as muscle contraction occurs.

Actin: The protein that forms the thinner myofilament, which consists of two strands of actin in a double helix configuration. As mentioned, the sarcomere contracts when actin and myosin (the thick filament) bind together and complete a power stroke.

Troponin: Troponin, a protein located at regular intervals along the actin filament, binds with the Ca^{2+} released from the sarcoplasmic reticulum. This causes a conformational change in tropomyosin, exposing the binding site on the actin filaments for the myosin heads to form cross-bridges.

Tropomyosin: Tropomyosin is a protein in the I-band located along the actin filament in a groove formed by the double helix configuration of the two actin strands. The conformational change of troponin moves the tropomyosin deeper into the groove, allowing the actin and myosin cross-bridge to rapidly attach, pulling the actin toward the center of sarcomere in a contractile action. When troponin is not affecting tropomyosin (i.e., no Ca^{2+} release), it inhibits actin and myosin bonding, which prevents a constant state of muscle contraction.

Acetylcholine (ACh): Vesicles located at the terminal end of motor neurons release the neurotransmitter ACh when an action potential arrives at the terminal end of a motor neuron. ACh diffuses across the synaptic space of the neuromuscular junction, and this excites the sarcolemma, initiating muscle contraction.

Muscular Dynamics Involved During Movement Patterns

<u>Sliding Filament Theory</u>
The sliding filament theory states that muscle shortening and lengthening is due to the movement of actin and myosin sliding past each other and reducing the distance between the Z-lines of the sarcomere because the overlap of the filaments increases. As the myosin cross-bridges attach and detach from actin filaments, the muscle fiber shortens due to the contractile action. Because minimal calcium is in the myofibril under resting conditions (during *resting phase*), very few myosin cross-bridges are bound with actin (i.e., actomyosin protein complex) because the binding sites are blocked. During the *excitation-contraction coupling phase*, the muscle releases an electrical discharge, and this starts a series of chemical events on the surface of the muscle cell, causing the release of calcium inside the muscle cell from the sarcoplasmic reticulum. The Ca^{2+} binds with troponin, resulting in tropomyosin moving farther into the double helix groove, allowing rapid binding of actin and myosin filaments and the power stroke that pulls the actin toward the center of the sarcomere. During the contraction phase, the enzyme myosin adenosine triphosphatase (ATPase) breaks down ATP into adenosine diphosphate (ADP). The ADP on the myosin cross-bridge globular head is replaced with ATP so that myosin head has energy to detach from the actin and then re-cock and grab on to the next binding spot on the actin filament, helping to "slide" down and create the sarcomere shortening needed for muscular contraction. If ATP and Ca^{2+} are still available, the entire contraction process (i.e., Ca^{2+} binds to troponin, myosin cross-bridge binds with actin, power stroke causes sarcomere contraction, actin and myosin uncouple, myosin head position is reset) is repeated in the muscle fiber during the *recharge phase*. Relaxation occurs when Ca^{2+}, ATP, ADP, or ATPase is no longer available. The *relaxation phase* also occurs when motor neurons stop releasing ACh, the Ca^{2+} levels in the sarcoplasmic reticulum return to baseline, and myosin and actin uncouple.

<u>All-or-None Principle</u>
This principle states that when an action potential in a motor neuron reaches the sarcolemma, the action potential will either elicit activation of all the muscle fibers connected to the motor neuron or no activation of any of the muscle fibers will occur. Partial activation of just some fibers will not occur.

<u>Types of Muscle Action</u>
Concentric muscle action: This type of action occurs when the contraction force is greater than the resistive force (F_r), causing the muscle to shorten. The tension caused by the shortening of the muscle causes the joint to move. When an athlete is doing biceps curls, the elbow is initially extended. The concentric action of the biceps results in the shortening of the muscle, moving the elbow to a flexed position.

Eccentric muscle action: When the external resistance is greater than the muscle force (F_M), the muscle develops tension and lengthens. During a biceps curl, the lowering of the weight when moving the arm from a flexed to extended position reflects the lengthening of the muscle, resulting from eccentric action.

Isometric muscle action: This results when a muscle generates force and attempts to contract concentrically, but is unable to because the resistance force is greater than that generated by the muscle. In this situation, the action does not cause movement or external work, but it does generate force. If an athlete is holding a fixed bar with elbows extended and attempts a concentric action to shorten the bicep, the biceps produces force, but movement does not occur (i.e., there is no change in the length of muscle fibers).

Isokinetic muscle action: Isokinetic muscle actions do not occur naturally by result in a dynamic movement performed at a constant velocity. For the muscle movement to occur at a constant velocity, a machine, such as a dynamometer (a device that allows constant velocity movement regardless of the amount of torque), must be used.

Neuromuscular Anatomy

Motor unit: The functional unit of the neuromotor system consisting of the motor neuron and all the muscle fibers it innervates. Motor unit function depends on the morphological and physiological characteristics of the muscle fibers innervated by the motor neuron.

Motor neuron (nerve cell): Consists of an alpha motor neuron (cell body), axon, and dendrites, the motor neuron transmits nerve impulses from the spinal cord to the muscle fiber. A myelin sheath surrounds the axon, with nodes interrupting the myelin every 1-2 millimeters. The alternation of myelin and nodes allows an electrical current (i.e., nerve impulse) to quickly move down the axon with impulses "jumping" from node to node. The terminal branches end at the neuromuscular junction.

Neuromuscular junction (AKA motor end plate): This is the functional connection (chemical synapse) between the end of the myelinated motor neuron and the muscle fiber. It transmits the nerve impulse from the motor neuron to the muscle fiber, initiating the stimulation of the nerve fiber by chemical transmission. The action potential reaches the terminal branches, and ACh is released across the synaptic space, stimulating the sarcolemma. When enough ACh is released, an action potential is generated and travels the length of the muscle fiber, causing it to contract.

Muscle spindles: Muscle spindles are proprioceptors that sense the rate and magnitude of increases in muscle tension as the muscle lengthens with an eccentric muscle contraction. The spindles contain *intrafusal fibers*, modified muscle fibers, contained in a sheath of connective tissue that runs parallel to the normal *extrafusal muscle fibers*. As a muscle lengthens, the muscle spindles are stretched, activating a sensory neuron in the spindle that sends an impulse to the spinal cord. In the spinal cord, the signal coming from the sensory neuron synapses with a motor neurons, which travels back to innervate the extrafusal muscle fibers. Motor neurons activate the muscle, causing a reflexive muscle action called the stretch reflex. This causes muscle contraction, the spindles shorten, and the sensory impulses stop. Increasing loads cause the spindles to stretch more. The muscle force (F_M) and power are potentiated by this reflexive contraction.

Golgi tendon organs (GTOs): These mechanoreceptors lie parallel to extrafusal muscle fibers near the musculotendinous junction and detect tension changes in an active muscle, acting as feedback monitors. The increased tension caused by muscle shortening stimulates GTOs to relax the muscle via the inhibitory interneuron; this response is also called autogenic inhibition. Reciprocal inhibition occurs when a contracting muscle stimulates the GTOs, causing the opposing muscle to relax. The GTOs respond to muscle tension by sending impulses to the spinal cord to elicit reflex inhibition. Importantly, GTOs protect the muscle and tendon from injury caused by an excessive load by prohibiting excessive tension to build up in a muscle. Stimulation of GTOs is graded based on the amount of tension a muscle develops, such that at low forces, the effect of GTOs is minimal, but with increasing loads, the GTOs mediate more significant reflexive inhibition.

Somatic nervous system: The somatic nervous system innervates skeletal muscles and is responsible for conscious control of voluntary movements.

Autonomic nervous system (ANS): The ANS innervates smooth and cardiac muscles, as well as glands. It is also responsible for visceral motor actions (e.g., pumping the heart, food movement through the digestive tract). The ANS, sometimes called the involuntary nervous system, is not under conscious control. It has two subdivisions: the sympathetic and parasympathetic nervous systems.

- Sympathetic nervous system (SNS): The SNS prepares the body for action and is sometimes called the fight-or-flight system. During exercise, the SNS is responsible for directing blood away from the digestive tract and skin and toward the skeletal muscles, heart, and brain. Physiological responses associated with the SNS include increased blood pressure (BP), heart rate, and blood glucose levels; sweating; and dilation of the pupils and lung bronchioles.

- Parasympathetic nervous system (PNS): The PNS is considered the "resting and digestion system" because its primary function is conserving body energy by maintaining body activities at baseline levels. The PNS is responsible for digestive tract motility, smooth muscle activity associated with urination and defecation, pupil constriction, and gland secretion.

Types of Muscle

Smooth Muscle has spindle-shaped fibers that are shorter and narrower than skeletal muscle fibers. Smooth muscle fibers only contain one nucleus and do not have striations. Sheets of these muscle fibers form the walls of blood vessels and the hollow organs of the urinary, digestive, respiratory, and reproductive tracts. The contraction and relaxation of smooth muscle is responsible for peristalsis, which moves substances through the digestive tract

Cardiac Muscle is only located in the wall of the heart and its contraction pumps blood through the heart and the body's blood vessels.

Skeletal Muscle is primarily used in the movement of bones at joints and for maintaining posture.

Muscle Fiber Types
Type I muscle fibers: Also known as slow-twitch muscle fibers (slow-oxidative fibers), metabolically, these fibers have a large capacity for aerobic energy supply and are relatively resistant to fatigue. Type I fibers have a limited ability to rapidly generate force because of their low anaerobic capacity and low myosin ATPase activity. Compared to Type II fibers, Type I muscle fibers have slower calcium-handling abilities, contract more slowly, have reduced glycolytic capacity, and they have numerous and relatively large mitochondria. Type I muscle fibers play an important role in endurance sports that rely on a sustained energy supply, such as long distance running (e.g., 5000 meters, marathon), soccer, cross-country skiing, and distance cycling and swimming.

Type IIa muscle fibers: Also known as fast-twitch muscle fibers, these fibers are energy inefficient, easily fatigable, and have low aerobic power. Type IIa fibers have a moderate capacity for both anaerobic and aerobic energy production. These fibers can be classified as fast-oxidative/glycolytic fibers, and they can rapidly generate force due to high myosin ATPase activity and anaerobic power. Type IIa fibers are surrounded by a greater number of capillaries than Type IIx fibers, allowing for greater aerobic metabolism.

Type IIx muscle fibers: Also a type of fast-twitch muscle fiber (sometimes called Type IIb fibers), Type IIx fibers have less capacity for aerobic energy production, making them more fatigable than Type IIa fibers. Type IIx fibers, considered to be fast-glycolytic (FG) fibers, have the greatest capacity for anaerobic energy production and the fastest shortening velocity so they can generate significant force.

Note that many sports (e.g., rowing, tennis, boxing, wrestling, soccer) require both Type I and Type II muscle fibers.

Types of Musculature Structures

Skeletal muscles vary in shape and function because of the various arrangements of the muscle fascicles. The table below provides the name of the fascicular arrangements, the structure of the fascicles, and an example of a muscle having each fascicular arrangement.

Name of Fascicular Arrangement	Structure of Fascicular Arrangement	Muscle Example
Circular	Fascicles are arranged in a concentric ring	Obicularis oris (muscles surrounding mouth)
Convergent (sometimes called radiate)	Muscle has a broad origin and is fan- or triangular-shaped	Pectoralis major; gluteus medius
Parallel/longitudinal	Long axis of fascicles are parallel to long axis of muscle.	Rectus abdominis
Unipennate	Short fascicles insert obliquely into only one side of tendon	Extensor digitorum longus; tibialis posterior
Bipennate	Fascicles insert into opposite sides of one central tendon	Rectus femoris
Multipennate	Tendon branches within the muscle	Deltoid
Fusiform	Spindle-shaped muscles	Biceps brachii

Here's an illustration of this:

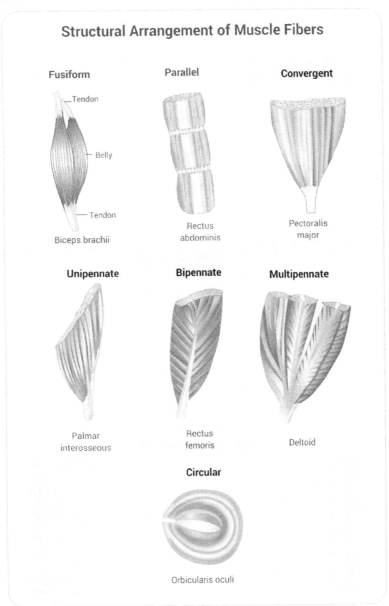

Structural Arrangement of Muscle Fibers

Fusiform
Tendon
Belly
Tendon
Biceps brachii

Parallel
Rectus abdominis

Convergent
Pectoralis major

Unipennate
Palmar interosseous

Bipennate
Rectus femoris

Multipennate
Deltoid

Circular
Orbicularis oculi

Neuromuscular Responses to Exercise

Motor Unit Recruitment Patterns
Motor units contain only one type of muscle fiber (i.e., Type I, Type IIa, Type IIx). The ability to produce force is a requirement in all sport activities. There are two ways that motor units modulate force production: summation and size principle.

Summation
Summation is dependent upon how frequently motor units are activated. A single activation will cause a minimal muscle twitch with little force production, but if that motor unit continues to be activated at a greater frequency, there can be a summative effect of these twitches, resulting in greater force production.

Size Principle

The second method used to modulate force production is dependent upon how many motor units are activated. If greater force is needed for an activity, more motor units will be recruited. This phenomenon, called the *size principle*, describes the interrelationship between force, motor unit recruitment thresholds, and firing rates. Smallest motor units are recruited first, and as more force is needed, larger motor units (that innervate more muscle fibers) are activated. Ascending recruitment of smaller to larger motor allows the continuum of low- to high-force production and smooth muscle movements when force changes, while conserving energy.

Selective Recruitment

This is an exception to the size principle. Under some circumstances, trained athletes can inhibit the activation of small motor units. This allows larger motor units to be activated immediately when rapid force production (e.g., vertical jump) is needed.

Nerve Conduction

When the electrical nerve impulse from the motor neuron arrives at the motor junction, ACh is released, converting the impulse into a chemical stimulus. This generates an action potential – a wave of depolarization – that travels the length of the muscle fiber through the T-tubules, causing the release of Ca^{2+}, which initiates the series of events leading to the contractile movement of the actin and myosin filaments.

Electromyography (EMG)

Surface and intramuscular EMG is used to assess the quality and quantity of the electrical activity within skeletal muscles resulting from neural activation by motor units. Greater neural activation is implicated when there is an increase in EMG signal.

Kinematic Principles of Movement

Anatomical Position

The position where a person is standing with arms at the side and the palms of the hands facing forward. From this position, the body can be divided into three anatomical planes that cut the body into sections. These anatomical planes are important because they can be used to explain normal and athletic movements and the type of resistance exercises for training these movements.

Sagittal plane: This plane divides the body into right and left regions. Examples of body movements and related exercises that occur in the sagittal plane are provided below.

Body Movement	Example Sport/Activity That Utilizes the Movement	Related Exercise
Elbow extension	Shot put	Triceps push-down
Hip flexion	Football punter	Leg raises
Knee flexion	Diving (tuck dive)	Leg curl

Frontal plane: The frontal plane runs through the center of the body from side to side, dividing the body into front and back halves.

Body Movement	Example Sport/Activity That Utilizes the Movement	Related Exercise
Shoulder adduction	Swimming (breaststroke)	Wide-grip lateral pull-down
Ankle inversion	Resisted inversion	Soccer dribbling
Hip adduction	Standing adduction machine	Soccer side step

Transverse plane: The transverse plane is a horizontal plane that divides the body into upper and lower regions.

Body Movement	Example Sport/Activity That Utilizes the Movement	Related Exercise
Hip internal rotation	Basketball pivot movement	Resisted internal rotation
Lower back left rotation	Baseball batting	Medicine ball side toss
Lower back right rotation	Golf swing	Torso machine

Joint Angle

A joint angle is the angle, measured in degrees, between two body parts that are linked by a single joint. Body movements occur due to rotation around a joint or multiple joints with the force produced expressed as torque. Torque exerted varies by joint due to various characteristics of the joint (e.g., range of motion [ROM]; the relationship of muscle length versus force; leverage resulting from the use of joints as first-, second-, and third-class levers; and speed of contraction of muscles at the joint).

Kinetic Laws and Principles of Movement

Velocity

Velocity is the rate of change of distance over time. Velocity and speed are often used interchangeably, but it is important for the strength and conditioning professional to separate the terms. Speed is the rate at which an object covers a distance, and velocity describes how fast and in what direction an object is moving. Velocity is calculated by dividing the distance traveled by the amount of time it took to cover that distance.

Force

Force is best visualized as a push or pull exerted on one object by a second object. It is the interaction of two physical objects that have both size (magnitude) and direction. Force is measured in Newtons (N) and can be calculated using the formula: $F = m(a + g)$; where F is force, m is the mass of a dumbbell or other object, a is instantaneous acceleration, and g is acceleration resulting from gravity (9.81 meters/second/second). The number of cross-bridges formed between actin and myosin filaments determines the amount of force produced at any moment in time.

Force-Velocity Curve

The force-velocity curve graphically represents the relationship between velocity (meters/second), plotted on the x-axis, and force (N), plotted on the y-axis. The curve shows the inverse relationship between force and velocity, such that as force increases, velocity decreases, and vice versa. The strength and conditioning professional must understand this relationship when planning a training program. For example, if an athlete is strong but not fast, more time should be spent training at a lower force intensity (e.g., back squats at 30 percent of one-repetition maximum [1RM] instead of at 90 percent of 1RM) and faster velocity to improve speed.

Force-Time Curve

The force-time curve graphically represents the relationship between time (milliseconds), plotted on the x-axis, and force, plotted on the y-axis.

Rate of force development (RFD): The RFD is the change in force divided by the change in time. It has significant relevance for sports where the timing of movements or explosiveness is critical. The generation of maximum force in minimum time is an index of explosive strength.

Momentum

Momentum is the amount of motion that an object has. It is calculated as the velocity multiplied by the object's mass, and like velocity, momentum is a vector quantity with a direction. Momentum is relevant to sports because it can be used for performance assessment. For example, an athlete having a mass of 125 kilograms and running at 10 meters/second will have more momentum than an athlete running at the same velocity who is 100 kilograms. Momentum can also play a role in injuries, particularly in collision sports (e.g., rugby, American football) because athletes having a large mass can hit or tackle another athlete with more momentum than athletes with less mass moving at the same speed.

Impulse

Impulse is the product of the time required to generate a force. This quantity is represented as the area under the force-time curve. Impulse increases by improving the RFD with the magnitude of change in the momentum of an object being contingent upon impulse.

Work

Work, measured in Joules [J], is calculated as the applied force on an object multiplied by the distance that the object is displaced (in the direction the force is applied). Quantifying work is useful for strength and conditioning programs because an athlete's training volume over the course of a training session, day, week, or the entire season can provide information about how well the athlete can handle varying amounts of training volume and intensity.

Work = Force × Displacement

Power

Power is the rate that work is performed and it can be calculated as work divided by time. Power can also be calculated as the product of force applied to an object and velocity. Power is usually measured in watts (W), but it can also be measured in horsepower (hp). Power must be considered, in addition to work, when designing a strength and conditioning program. Training should consider the power associated with an athlete's sport or activity, and it should use various power outputs relevant to sport-specific movement velocities. Because power is the product of force and velocity, improving either of these components will improve the athlete's RFD and explosiveness.

Power = Work/Time

Center of Gravity (COG)

The balance point of an object when torque is equal on all sides is the COG. The COG is also the point where the planes of the body intersect. From a sports perspective, the lower an athlete's COG, the more stability he or she has. For example, hockey players skating with flexed knees low over the puck have increased stability, making it more difficult for opponents to get the player off of the puck.

Center of Pressure (COP)

COP refers to the point of application of ground reaction force, which is the force that is exerted by the supporting surface (e.g., ground) on the body. COP is relevant for postural control and gait and contributes to balance and stability. A tennis player may shift his or her COP medially and laterally as seen when the player moves from side to side before receiving a serve.

Musculoskeletal Lever Systems

Levers

Levers are rigid or semi-rigid bodies that pivot on a fixed point or fulcrum, and when F_M is applied (i.e., effort), the lever moves a load (i.e., resistive force [F_r]). Joints act as the body's fulcrums when bones and muscle interact. Muscle contraction provides the force required to move an object against a resistive force. The load consists of the bone, the tissue over the bone, and whatever load is being moved. The three types of levers differ based on the relative position of three elements: F_M, F_r, and the fulcrum. Levers are relevant to sport activities because they allow a specific amount of effort to move a heavier load or to move a load farther or faster than would otherwise be possible. The majority of muscles in the body operate as third-class levers.

Joints

Joints are the junctions between bones that control movement. *Fibrous joints*, such as those in the skull, allow almost no movement, whereas *cartilaginous joints*, such as intervertebral joints, allow a limited amount of movement. *Synovial joints*, such as the elbow, allow the greatest amount of movement and ROM. Sport and exercise movements primarily occur around synovial joints (see the table below for specific synovial joints) because of the ROM and reduced friction that they afford.

Synovial Joint Type	Movements	Examples
Ball-and-socket	Rotation and movement in all planes	Hip, shoulder
Condylar	No rotation; variety of movements in different planes	Joints between phalanges and metacarpals
Plane	Twisting or sliding	Joints between various bones of the ankle and wrist
Hinge	Flexion and extension	Elbow
Pivot	Rotation	Joint between the proximal ends of the ulna and radius
Saddle	Variety of movements; primarily in two planes	Joint between carpal and metacarpal of thumb

Joints can also be classified based on the type of movement they allow, specifically, the number of directions that joint rotation can occur. A uniaxial joint, such as the elbow, rotates around only one axis and operates as a hinge. The wrist and ankle are examples of biaxial joints, which allow movement around two perpendicular axes. Multiaxial joints, such as the shoulder and hip joint, allow movement around three axes (any direction in space).

Fulcrum: The fixed pivot point of a lever.

Muscle force (FM): The force generated by the contraction of a muscle.

Resistive force (FR): An external source of resistance (e.g., gravity, friction, weights, inertia) that counters the action of the F_r.

Torque: Also called moment, torque is the extent that a force tends to rotate an object around a specific fulcrum. Muscles pull on bones to create movement, maintain body position, and resist movement, and this force acts on the bones (levers) at the joints. Torque can be quantified as the magnitude of the force multiplied by the length of the moment arm and is measured in Newton meters (N·m).

Moment arm: Also called the lever arm, force arm, or torque arm, the moment arm is the perpendicular distance from the line of action (i.e., the long line that passes through the point where force is applied in the direction of the force exerted) of the force to the fulcrum.

Mechanical advantage: It is the trade-off of distance and force, because it is the ratio of the moment arm through which an applied force acts (i.e., F_M) through the F_r.

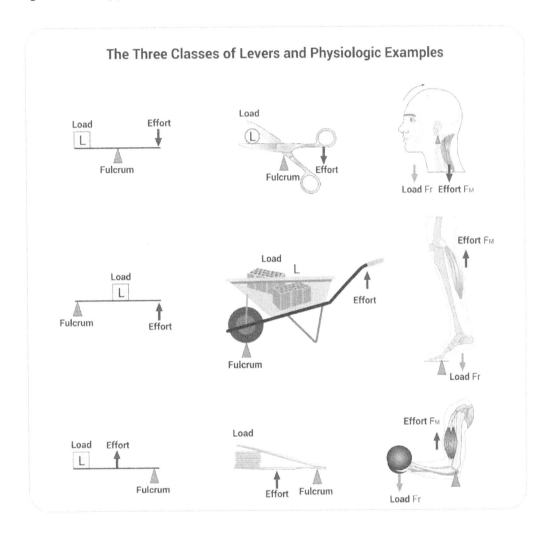

First-class lever: (e.g., a seesaw) has the F_M applied at one end of the lever; the F_r is at the other end with the fulcrum located somewhere in the middle (i.e., F_r → fulcrum → F_M). The forearm can serve as a first-class lever during triceps extension exercises. The fulcrum is the elbow joint; F_M comes from the contraction of the triceps, and the F_r is the weight machine.

Second-class lever: Consists of a fulcrum at one end, the F_M is applied to the other end, and the F_r is between the ends (i.e., fulcrum → F_r → F_M). A wheelbarrow is a second-class lever. The wheel is the fulcrum, the F_r is the load in the wheelbarrow, and the F_M is applied to the handles. An example of a second-class lever in the body is standing on one's toes. The metatarsophalangeal joints act as the fulcrum, body weight is the load, and the calf muscle provides the effort as it pulls up on the heel.

Third-class lever: F_r is at one end of the lever, F_M is applied in the middle of the lever, and the fulcrum is at the other end (i.e., F_r → F_M →fulcrum). A biceps curl is an example of a third-class lever; the F_r is the barbell, F_M is the contraction of the biceps, and the fulcrum is the elbow joint.

Role of Muscles and Movement

Agonist
A muscle, or group of muscles, that is most directly responsible for generating the force to produce a movement; it is also called a prime mover. When lowering the body in the downward phase of a squat, the agonists are the gluteus maximus and the quadriceps group.

Antagonist
Antagonists generate a motion or force that is the opposite of the agonist's motion. Sometimes an antagonist is a muscle, or muscle groups, that performs a protective action, such as decelerating a force acting on the body or helping stabilize working joints.

Synergist
A muscle that indirectly helps to generate force production during a movement or one that aids in stabilizing the agonist muscle as force is produced.

Neutralizer
Neutralizers prevent unwanted or extraneous movement by pulling against and canceling out the motion from the agonist. For example, when the elbow is flexed, supination is often undesirable, so the pronator teres counteracts the supination of the biceps so that only elbow flexion results.

Stabilizer
Also called a fixator, a muscle acting as a stabilizer muscle holds certain joints or body segments immobile, so that agonists can optimize movement and force production. For example, to do an abdominal exercise, the pelvis may be stabilized by the contraction of the muscles of the hip joint. It is often optimal to hold the insertion point or proximal joint stable, so that the working muscles have a more fixed end to pull from.

The muscles involved in the flexion of the forearm at the elbow joint and their roles in the movement are provided in the table below.

Muscle	Movement Role
Biceps brachii	Agonist (prime mover)
Triceps brachii	Antagonist
Deltoid	Stabilizer (fixator)
Brachioradialis	Neutralizer

Bone and Connective Tissue Anatomy

Bones
The human skeleton has approximately 206 bones and these bones provide protection and support for the body. Bones can be divided into the *axial* (skull, vertebral column, sternum, and ribs) and *appendicular* (the right and left clavicle and scapula and the left and right bones of the arm, forearm, and hand; the left and right coaxial and the left and right bones of the leg and foot) *skeletons.* Bones

consist of varying amounts of spongy (*trabecular*) and compact (*cortical*) bone. A shell of dense cortical bone surrounds interlocking columns of trabecular bone called osteons. Bone marrow – composed of adipose tissue, vasculature, and the manufacturing site of blood vessels – occupies the space between the trabeculae and blood vessels and extends from the marrow cavity to cortical bone. *Bone periosteum*, connective tissue that covers all bones, is attached to tendons.

Collagen
Collagen is the primary structural component of all connective tissue. Bones, ligaments, and tendons are Type I collagen, and cartilage is composed of Type 2 collagen. Both types of collagen are formed from procollagen molecules, which consist of three protein strands in a triple helix formation. An enzyme produces active collagen, which aligns with other collagen molecules to form long filaments that are the components of microfibrils that form bundles as bone grows. The strength and durability of collagen stems from strong cross-linking bonds, formed between adjacent collagen bundles. The longitudinal grouping of these bundles together forms ligaments and tendons. The bundles can also be arranged in layered sheets of varying directions, as found in fascia, bone, and cartilage.

Tendons and Ligaments
Tendons are fibrous connective tissue connecting muscle to the periosteum of bone. Muscle contractions pull the tendon, causing the attached bone to move. Ligaments are fibrous connective tissue connecting bone to bone. Ligaments contain elastin, a type of elastic protein that provides the stretch needed for normal joint movement. Tendons and ligaments contain relatively few cells that require little oxygen and nutrients for metabolic activity. Because of the limited vasculature and circulation in tendons, regeneration after injury takes a significant amount of time and is sometimes not possible without surgical intervention.

Bone and Connective Tissue Responses to Exercise and Training

Bone
Anaerobic Training
Minimal essential strain (MES) is the stimulus threshold required to initiate new bone growth. Anaerobic training can stimulate bone growth and should utilize specificity of loading and progressive overload to do so. Specificity of loading requires the use of specific movement patterns and exercises that directly load the targeted growth region of the athlete's skeleton. Exercises should involve multiple joints and apply increasingly heavier external loads. The anaerobic exercise components of mechanical load that stimulate bone growth are the intensity of the load, the speed of loading, the direction of the force, and the volume of the loading. Bone deposition follows Wolff's Law, which states that bone remodels according to the forces placed upon it; if forces are sufficient in intensity and frequency, bones become stronger, building additional matrix and mineralization, or they atrophy and thin with disuse.

Aerobic Training
Aerobic programs that stimulate bone growth must be high-intensity weight-bearing activities (e.g., running, aerobics). The intensity of activity has to increase progressively to ensure continual overload of the bone. Because bone responds to the intensity and rate of external loading, when it is no longer possible to increase activity intensity, increasing the rate of the limb movement is required. This can be achieved with high-intensity interval training (HIIT).

Connective Tissue

Anaerobic Training
High-intensity anaerobic training causes connective tissue growth and structural changes. Increased enzyme activity, due to anaerobic training, results in the formation of collagen that aligns with other collagen molecules to form long filaments. Specific changes within a tendon include an increase in collagen fibril diameter, number, and packing density. These adaptations increase the tensional forces that the tendon can withstand. Anaerobic training increases tendon stiffness, which is directly associated with muscular recoil and power production – an important component of performance in some sports.

Aerobic Training
Similar to bone, aerobic exercise intensity that exceeds the strain put on connective tissue during normal activities is required for connective tissue changes to occur.

Characteristics of the Energy Systems

Bioenergetics
Bioenergetics refers to the flow of energy within a biological system and is primarily focused on how macronutrients, containing chemical energy, from food (i.e., carbohydrates, proteins, fats) are converted into biologically usable forms of energy to perform work.

Catabolism
Catabolism is the process of breaking large molecules into smaller molecules to make energy available to the organism. For example, carbohydrates are catabolized to provide fuel for exercise and normal physiological processes. Catabolism also can involve the breakdown of muscle tissue during periods of heavy training volume, low caloric intake, or high stress.

Anabolism
Anabolism is the process of restructuring or building larger compounds from catabolized materials, such as assembling amino acids into structural proteins, which are needed to maintain homeostasis and to generate new muscle tissue.

Exergonic Reaction
Exergonic reaction are chemical reactions that result in the release of energy from the system, which can then be used to perform work. These reactions are spontaneous and favorable.

Endergonic Reaction
A type of chemical reaction that requires the input of energy. In the body, this energy comes in the form of adenosine triphosphate (ATP). These reactions are not spontaneous and are typically involved with anabolic processes.

Metabolism
Metabolism is the sum total of all catabolic and anabolic reactions occurring in the human body. Essential physiological processes such as muscle growth and hormone balance rely on these reactions and continually occur so that the body can maintain homeostasis. It is possible to evaluate an athlete's energy expenditure (metabolic rate) and fitness level using direct or indirect calorimetry.

Adenosine Triphosphate (ATP)
ATP is a high-energy molecule used for muscle contractions, movement, and other life-sustaining metabolic processes. ATP is an intermediate molecule (consisting of three primary parts—an adenine, a

ribose, and three phosphates in a chain) that allows energy to transfer from exergonic to endergonic and catabolic to anabolic reactions. ATP is generated and replenished in skeletal muscles by three energy systems: phosphagen, glycolytic, and oxidative.

ATP Hydrolysis
Hydrolysis is a general term for any chemical reaction that breaks a chemical bond via the addition of water. ATP hydrolysis splits the ATP molecule into adenosine diphosphate (ADP) and usable energy. The enzyme adenosine triphosphatase (ATPase) is the catalyst for the hydrolysis of ATP. The following equation shows the reactants (left of arrow), enzyme (middle), and products (right of arrow) for ATP hydrolysis:

$$\text{ATP} + \text{H}_2\text{O} \leftarrow \text{ATPASE} \rightarrow \text{ADP} + \text{P}_i + \text{H}^+ + \text{Energy}$$

Adenosine Diphosphate (ADP)
When ATP undergoes hydrolysis, ADP (containing two phosphate groups), an inorganic phosphate molecule, a hydrogen ion, and free energy are produced.

ATPase
ATPase is the enzyme responsible for catalyzing the breakdown of ATP to ADP. The dephosphorylation reaction results in the release of energy used to carry out other chemical reactions.

Myosin ATPase
Myosin ATPase catalyzes ATP hydrolysis, providing the energy for cross-bridge recycling.

Calcium ATPase
Calcium ATPase is the enzyme that provides the energy used to regulate calcium movement by pumping it into the sarcoplasmic reticulum.

Sodium-Potassium ATPase
This enzyme controls the sodium potassium concentration gradient in the sarcolemma after depolarization to maintain the cellular resting potential. For every two K^+ ions pumped into the cell, there are three NA^+ ions pumped out.

Adenosine Monophosphate (AMP)
AMP results from ADP hydrolysis, which cleaves the second phosphate group, leaving one.

Biological Energy Systems
There are several basic biological energy systems in muscle cells that replace ATP. The phosphagen and glycolytic systems occur in the sarcoplasm and are anaerobic mechanisms, which means that they do not require oxygen. The electron transport chain (ETC) and Krebs cycle are aerobic mechanisms that require oxygen and occur in the mitochondria. The cellular respiration systems act in concert, rather than individually, to provide all required energy during exercise or rest.

Phosphagen System (ATP-phosphocreatine [PC])

The phosphagen system utilizes ATP hydrolysis for high-intensity activities of short length (e.g., resistance training; short, intense sprints; other vigorous bouts up to about 10 seconds in duration) and is also active at the start of all types of exercise of varying intensities until the other systems have had time to start producing energy. This system relies on the breakdown of creatine phosphate (CP) for energy. Because ATP stores are quickly depleted and ATP is required for cellular functions other than muscle contractions, the phosphagen system uses CP stores to maintain ATP concentrations. This system is rapidly depleted after about 10 seconds of maximal intensity work, so the glycolytic system starts to engage and contribute energy after this point. It takes longer for glycolysis, and especially oxidative energy systems, to generate energy, which is why the phosphagen system is the initial source.

Creatine Phosphate (CP)

CP, also called phosphocreatine (PC), concentrations in muscles are four to six times greater than ATP muscle stores, with higher CP concentrations in Type II muscle fibers. The phosphagen system uses creatine kinase in the chemical reaction that combines a phosphate group from CP with ADP to replenish ATP. CP is stored in small amounts, limiting the phosphagen system to supplying energy for intense, short bouts of exercise.

$$ADP + CP \leftarrow \text{Creatine kinase} \rightarrow ATP + \text{Creatine}$$

Creatine Kinase

Creatine kinase is the enzyme required to catalyze the reaction that combines ADP and CP to form ATP and creatine. Elevated levels of creatine kinase in blood serum tests are an indicator of muscle damage (e.g., kidney failure, heart attack). In athletes, too much work performed in a training session (single or aggregate sessions) can cause rhabdomyolysis, the rapid breakdown of muscles, elevating levels of creatine kinase in blood serum.

Adenylate Kinase

Also called myokinase, this enzyme catalyzes a reaction that replenishes ATP.

$$2ADP \leftarrow \text{adenylate kinase} \rightarrow ATP + AMP$$

Law of Mass Action/Mass Action Effect

This law states that the concentration of reactants, products, or both in solution will influence the direction of the reactions. These are often referred to as near-equilibrium reactions because they continue in the given direction based on the concentration of available reactants. This equilibrium is specific to the amount of ATP needed for the specific work being completed by the athlete. The reactions will continue until the exercise intensity is low enough for another energy system to take over or the exercise ends.

Glycolytic System

Glycolysis

Glycolysis is the breakdown of glucose to replenish ATP. Glucose either comes directly out of blood circulation or is broken down from glycogen stores in the muscles or liver, or is converted from other substrates. ATP replenished during glycolysis is slower than the replenishment provided by the single-step phosphagen system because glycolysis has ten steps and actually requires an investment of energy to drive some of the early steps in the energy pathway. The glycolytic system has an advantage, as it can produce significantly more ATP because of the relatively large supply of glucose and glycogen in the body versus the limited supply of CP.

Anaerobic Glycolysis (Fast Glycolysis)

ATP is produced by breaking down glucose without oxygen available during glycolysis. This process relies on converting pyruvate to lactate to replace ATP during short, high-intensity activity lasting 2 minutes or less. In the absence of oxygen, pyruvate does not get shuttled to the mitochondria for the Krebs Cycle. Instead, the lactate accumulates and must be broken down in the muscle or shuttled to the liver where it undergoes the Cori cycle.

Pyruvate

Pyruvate is the result of anaerobic glycolysis; one glucose molecule produces two pyruvate molecules. Pyruvate can either be converted to lactate in the sarcoplasm or be transported to the mitochondria for the Krebs cycle. Compared to pyruvate conversion to lactate, the Krebs cycle takes longer to replenish ATP because there are more steps required in the reaction series. However, the Krebs cycle can continue for a longer duration when exercise intensity is low. This process is aerobic glycolysis (also called slow glycolysis).

Pyruvate conversion to lactate: The enzyme *lactate dehydrogenase* catalyzes the reaction converting pyruvate to lactate. Lactate produced by anaerobic glycolysis can be cleared by oxidation within the muscle fiber, or it can be moved to the liver via the blood and converted into glucose. The process of the liver turning lactate to glucose is referred to as the *Cori cycle*.

The net reaction of glycolysis when pyruvate is converted to lactate:

$$\text{Glucose} + 2P_i + 2ADP \rightarrow 2\text{Lactate} + 2ATP + H_2O$$

Pyruvate transported to mitochondria for Krebs cycle: If oxygen is available, pyruvate and two molecules of nicotinamide adenine dinucleotide (NADH) will be transported to the mitochondria. Pyruvate is converted to acetyl-coenzyme A (acetyl-CoA) by pyruvate dehydrogenase, resulting in the loss of carbon (CO_2), and enters the Krebs cycle to resynthesize ATP. The Krebs cycle, a continuation of the substrate oxidation from glycolysis, is a series of reactions that results in the production of two ATP molecules.

The net reaction for glycolysis when pyruvate is transported to the mitochondria:

$$\text{Glucose} + 2P_i + 2ADP + 2NAD^+ \rightarrow 2\text{Pyruvate} + 2ATP + 2NADH + 2H_2O$$

Phosphorylation

Phosphorylation is addition of an inorganic phosphate to a molecule. Phosphorylation of ADP to ATP occurs by adding a phosphoryl (PO_3) group to ADP.

Substrate-Level Phosphorylation

Substrate-level phosphorylation is a single enzyme-generated reaction that uses ADP to directly resynthesize ATP. It occurs during anaerobic glycolysis (fast phosphorylation) and can occur during both anaerobic and aerobic activities.

Oxidative Phosphorylation

This is the process of ATP being resynthesized via the actions of the ETC. The oxidative system produces approximately thirty-eight ATP molecules when a molecule of glucose is processed all the way through glycolysis, the Krebs cycle, and the ETC. The oxidative system produces approximately 90 percent of the ATP yield while substrate-level phosphorylation accounts for approximately the remaining 10 percent.

Electron Transport Chain (ETC)

In addition to two pyruvate molecules produced by glycolysis, six molecules of NADH and two molecules of flavin adenine dinucleotide ($FADH_2$) are produced and used by the ETC. Hydrogen atoms, transported by NADH and $FADH_2$ to the ETC, are used to produce ATP from ADP. The hydrogen atoms form a proton concentration gradient down the ETC that produces energy required to synthesize ATP. NADH and $FADH_2$ molecules rephosphorylate ADP to ATP via the ETC with each NADH molecule producing three ATP molecules and each $FADH_2$ producing two ATP molecules.

Oxidative System

During low-intensity activity and while the body is at rest, ATP is primarily supplied by the oxidative system, which utilizes carbohydrates and fats as substrates. Fats, compared to carbohydrates and proteins, have the greatest capacity for ATP production through their metabolism. The gross energy production of a molecule of glucose is 40 ATP and this number climbs to 463 ATP molecules for one 18-carbon triglyceride molecule. Protein is not a primary substrate and is only used for energy during long-duration exercise (more than 90 minutes) or times of starvation. During rest, approximately 70 percent of the ATP is produced from fat metabolism, and approximately 30 percent comes from the breakdown of carbohydrates. With the initiation of high-intensity activity, nearly 100 percent of ATP comes from carbohydrates metabolism. During long bouts of submaximal exercise, carbohydrates are used initially (due to their faster metabolism), but there is a slow shift back to using fats as glycogen stores deplete.

Net ATP Production
The net ATP production from the oxidation of one glucose molecule can be determined by adding the number of ATP molecules produced during each process. During glycolysis, substrate-level phosphorylation and oxidative phosphorylation produce four and six ATP molecules, respectively. During the Krebs cycle, substrate-level phosphorylation produces two ATP molecules, oxidative phosphorylation of eight NADH produces twenty-four ATP molecules, and the two $FADH_2$ molecules produce four ATP. These processes combined yield a total of forty ATP molecules. Two ATP molecules are used by glycolysis, so the net ATP production is thirty-eight ATP molecules.

Effects of Manipulating Training Variables to Target Specific Energy Systems

Interval training can be used to target any of the energy systems. To stress the *phosphagen system*, the maximum power should be 90-100 percent, with an exercise duration of 5-10 seconds and a work-to-rest ratio between 1:12 and 1:20. To emphasize the glycolytic pathway, 75-90 percent of maximum power is needed for 15-30 seconds with a work-to-rest ratio of 1:3 to 1:5. The combined targeting of the glycolytic and oxidative systems requires an exercise duration of 1-3 minutes at 30-75 percent of maximum power with a work-to-rest ratio of 1:3 to 1:4. To specifically target the oxidative system, a low percentage of maximal power (20-30 percent) is needed, but the duration of exercise needs to be greater than 3 minutes with a short work-to-rest ratio of 1:1 to 1:3.

Effect of Mode, Intensity, Duration, and Volume on Energy Systems
Strength and conditioning professionals must understand the activities required by an athlete to ensure the development of a training regimen that uses the appropriate mode, intensity, duration, and volume, while ultimately impacting energy system adaptations for specific sport activities. The use of relevant training intensities and rest intervals allows for the focus on a specific metabolic energy system during sessions to ultimately optimize performance.

High-intensity interval training (HIIT) uses brief bouts of high-intensity exercise followed by a recovery. HIIT typically uses running, cycling, resistance training, or calisthenics, and an HIIT program should be developed based on the specific goals of an individual athlete. Combining aerobic and anaerobic exercise is thought to enhance recovery.

Neuroendocrine Physiology

The organs and glands of the *endocrine system* release hormones that regulate physiological processes and maintain homeostasis when the body is confronted with external stimuli or environmental stressors such as altitude or exercise. The endocrine system releases hormones that regulate blood glucose levels, metabolism, tissue growth, recovery, reproduction, and mood. *Neuroendocrine physiology* refers to the interaction between the nervous and endocrine systems whereby hormones are released from glands receiving direct neural stimulation.

Functions of Hormones

Hormones are chemical messengers or signaling molecules produced by endocrine glands and other specific cells, which are created, stored, and released into the blood to stimulate specific physiological responses. Hormones are classified into three categories. Fat-soluble *steroid hormones* (e.g., cortisol, testosterone) passively diffuse across cell membranes and are responsible for primary and secondary sex characteristics, and are involved in metabolic control, immunity, fluid balance, and inflammation. *Polypeptide hormones* (e.g., insulin, growth hormones) are made of chains of amino acids inside the nucleus of cells. Because they are not fat-soluble, they serve as secondary messengers, signaling other hormones and hormonal cascades. *Amine hormones* consist of the amino acids tyrosine (e.g., dopamine, norepinephrine, epinephrine) and tryptophan (e.g., serotonin). Amine hormones bind to membrane receptors and work via secondary messengers. Hormones can also be categorized into *anabolic* and *catabolic*, where anabolic hormones promote tissue building and catabolic ones break down cellular components.

How Hormones Work

The *lock and key principle* refers to a binding mechanism of hormones and enzymes where the hormone receptor site has a specific structure that allows a single hormone to bind to the site, similar to a key fitting one specific lock. This principle is a simplistic view of hormone binding that does not take into account cross-reactivity, allosteric binding sites, or the need for the aggregation of several linked hormones to produce the optimal signal. *Cross-reactivity* occurs when a hormone fits the receptor but needs to interact with other hormones to produce a response. Some receptors have *allosteric binding sites* where substances other than the specific hormone can increase or decrease the response to the primary hormone via feedback loops.

Anabolic Hormones

Testosterone, growth hormone, and insulin-like growth factors are the primary anabolic hormones involved in muscle remodeling and growth.

Testosterone: Testosterone is the primary androgen (male sex hormone) in human physiology. Both males and females are affected by testosterone, although males have significantly higher levels of testosterone. Testosterone increases protein synthesis and the rate of cellular metabolism and red blood cell production. Testosterone is produced by the testes in males and the ovaries and adrenal glands in females.

Growth Hormone: The anterior pituitary gland secretes growth hormone, which has a significant influence on metabolism and energy availability. It is responsible for increasing the uptake of amino acids into skeletal muscle, and for increasing protein synthesis, facilitating the growth of Type I and Type II muscle fibers. Growth hormone has numerous other roles including decreasing glucose utilization and glycogen synthesis, increasing the availability of glucose and amino acids, increasing collagen synthesis and cartilage growth, and enhancing immune cell function.

Insulin-Like Growth Factors (IGFs): The majority of the growth-promoting effects of growth hormone are indirectly controlled by IGFs. These growth-promoting proteins are produced by skeletal muscle, bone, the liver, and other tissues. IGFs stimulate the uptake of amino acids from the blood to be used for cellular proteins and the uptake of sulfur needed for the cartilage matrix.

Hormones produced by the adrenal gland play a critical role in the fight-or-flight response and are also responsive to exercise stress. Cortisol and catecholamines are the adrenal hormones that are most important in exercise training.

Cortisol: Cortisol, a glucocorticoid secreted by the adrenal cortex, is a catabolic hormone in skeletal muscle; however, its principle role is to ensure that energy is available. It is a primary signaling hormone for carbohydrate metabolism and is associated with the storage of glycogen in muscle tissue. Cortisol increases the production of glucose in the liver and glycogen production in skeletal muscles. Overtraining can cause chronically high levels of cortisol, which can result in loss of strength and lean muscle mass.

Catecholamines: Epinephrine, norepinephrine, and dopamine are secreted by the adrenal medulla and have a significant role in many physiological functions. In muscle, epinephrine and norepinephrine increase muscle blood flow due to vasodilation, elevate blood pressure (BP), increase the rate of muscle contraction, increase energy availability, enhance metabolic enzyme activity, and increase testosterone secretion rates.

Neuroendocrine Responses to Exercise and Training

Anaerobic Responses
During anaerobic training, hormones have a variety of regulatory roles that impact homeostatic mechanisms tasked with keeping functions of the body within normal ranges during exercise and rest. There are four primary endocrine responses to anaerobic training:

1. Acute anabolic hormone responses to anaerobic exercise are crucial for both exercise performance and the resultant training adaptations. For up to 30 minutes after anaerobic resistance training, testosterone, growth hormone, and cortisol concentrations are elevated. Such changes generally occur rapidly and are quickly stabilized as the body responds to the homeostatic challenges associated with acute and long-term exercise training. Hormone levels are elevated most with resistance exercises that utilize large muscle groups or with moderate- to high-volume and -intensity exercises are combined with short rest intervals. The demands of acute anaerobic exercise cause increases in the concentration of catecholamines. Increased catecholamine concentrations are associated with the regulation of force production, energy availability, the rate of muscle contraction, and increased concentrations of testosterone and other hormones.

2. Chronic changes in acute hormonal responses: When an athlete participates in a long-term resistance training program, changes in endocrine function correspond to the increased exercise stress that the body is capable of handling. It is thought that any chronic adaptations in hormonal response patterns to acute anaerobic exercise may enhance the athlete's ability to handle and maintain higher-resistance exercise intensities for longer time periods.

3. Chronic changes in resting hormone concentrations after anaerobic exercise have not consistently been found with growth hormone, testosterone, or insulin-like growth factor. Resting-state hormone concentrations likely reflect factors such as muscle tissue response to intensity or volume changes in the resistance training program. The elevated concentrations of hormones after resistance training are great enough to influence muscle tissue remodeling, so increased resting concentrations of hormones are not necessary to facilitate training adaptations. Chronically high levels of anabolic steroids can be detrimental, causing downregulation (i.e., decreased number of receptors on target cell surface) of hormone receptors. Athletes using such performance enhancers try to combat this by cycling the drugs.

4. Hormone receptor changes have been shown to occur in response to resistance training. For example, androgen receptors seem to be upregulated within 48-72 hours after training. Changes in receptors mediate adaptations stimulated by hormonal responses.

Athletes can use resistance training to manipulate the endocrine system response and enhance training adaptations. For example, increasing the number of muscle fibers recruited for a resistance exercise increases the potential remodeling of the entire muscle.

Additionally, acute increases in serum testosterone concentrations can be achieved by using the following methods individually or in combination:

- Perform exercises such as squats, dead lift, and power clean, which target large muscles.
- Use heavy resistance loads that are 85-95 percent of one-repetition maximum (1RM).
- Performing multiple exercises or multiple sets to achieve moderate- to high-volume.
- Utilize short rest intervals of 30-60 seconds.

Growth hormone concentration levels can be increased acutely using one or both of the following training methods:

- Perform three sets of each exercise at high intensity with short (i.e., 1-minute) rest periods.
- Consume carbohydrates and protein before and after resistance training sessions.

Optimization of adrenal hormone responses can be achieved by the following method:

- Perform high-volume resistance exercises that utilize large muscles combined with short rest periods. This causes the body to experience adrenergic stress. Note that adequate rest and a varied training protocol should be utilized to avoid this stress leading to nonfunctional overreaching or overtraining.

Aerobic Responses
High-intensity aerobic training enhances the secretion of hormones in response to maximal aerobic exercise. This response likely improves the athlete's ability to handle and maintain high aerobic exercise intensities over long periods of time.

Cardiopulmonary Anatomy

Cardiovascular System
Heart Structures
The *heart* is a muscle called the *myocardium*. It has a left and a right *atrium*, which deliver blood to the left and right *ventricles*, respectively. Ventricle contraction produces the force necessary to eject blood out of the heart into circulation. The *tricuspid valve* and *mitral valve* form the atrioventricular (AV) valves. During ventricular contraction (*systole*), the AV valves prevent blood from flowing back from the ventricles into the atria. The *aortic valve* and the *pulmonary valve* form the *semilunar valves*. During ventricular relaxation (*diastole*), the semilunar valves prevent backflow from the aorta and pulmonary arteries into the ventricles.

Blood Pressure (BP)
Systole is the highest pressure and top number recorded in a BP reading. It represents the pressure exerted by the blood on the walls of the blood vessels. Systole occurs during the contractile phase of the cardiac cycle, which forces oxygen-rich blood into the body and blood into the pulmonary arteries to be

oxygenated in the lungs. During *diastole*, the heart chambers relax and fill with blood; this is the lowest pressure and bottom number in the BP measurement.

Electrical Conduction System
The mechanical contraction of the heart is controlled by an electrical conduction system. The conduction system has numerous components that are responsible for the transmission of the electrical impulse that causes the contraction and recovery of the atria and ventricles. The *sinoatrial (SA) node*, considered to be the intrinsic pacemaker, normally is the initiator of rhythmic electrical impulses. It consists of a small amount of specialized muscle tissue and is located in the upper wall of the right atrium. Internodal pathways conduct the electrical impulse between the SA node and *AV node*, which is the location where the electrical impulse is slightly delayed before it passes into the ventricles. The *AV bundle* conducts the electrical impulse to the ventricles and it is divided into left and a right bundle branches. The bundle branches are further divided into *Purkinje fibers*, which transmit the impulse throughout the ventricles.

Regulation of the Electrical Activity of the Heart
The autonomic nervous system (ANS) is responsible for the rhythmicity and conduction properties of the myocardium. The atria have both sympathetic and parasympathetic fibers, while the ventricles have mostly sympathetic fibers. Sympathetic fibers increase the speed at which the SA node depolarizes, resulting in a faster heart rate. Parasympathetic fibers decrease the speed of SA node depolarization, which decreases heart rate. The normal range for resting heart rate is 60-100 beats/minute. *Bradycardia* is an abnormally slow heart (less than 60 beats/minute), and *tachycardia* is an abnormally fast heart rate, defined as greater than 100 beats/minute.

Measuring the Electrical Activity of the Heart
An *electrocardiogram* (ECG) graphically represents the heart's electrical changes (recorded by electrodes on the skin) during the cardiac cycle. The cardiac cycle consists of several waves that represent depolarization and repolarization of the atria and ventricles. The first wave is the *P-wave*. This corresponds to atrial depolarization, which causes the contraction of the atria and the movement of blood down to the ventricles. The depolarization of the ventricles during the *QRS complex* (QRS complex consists of the *Q-wave*, *R-wave*, and *S-wave*) results in ventricular contraction, which produces the force to circulate blood through the pulmonary and peripheral blood vessels. The *T-wave* corresponds to ventricular repolarization, which can be thought of as the recovery from depolarization. The atria also repolarize, but this activity is masked on an EKG by the large QRS complex, which occurs simultaneously.

Vascular System: Arterial and Venous
The *arterial system* carries blood away from the heart, and blood returns to the heart via the *venous system*. Because *arteries* quickly move blood away from the heart with high pressure, they have strong, muscular walls. The arteries branch into *arterioles* that help to control the flow of blood into the *capillaries*. Arterioles have strong muscular walls that can constrict, closing completely, or become dilated, effectively controlling the flow of blood into the capillaries. Capillaries are the point of exchange for nutrients, hormones, oxygen, fluids, and electrolytes between the blood and the interstitial fluid of body tissues. Blood from the capillaries is collected by *venules* that converge into *veins* and return the blood to the heart. Unlike arteries, veins have thin but muscular walls that can dilate or constrict. Some veins in the leg have one-way valves to help ensure the one-way flow of blood and prevent backflow. The vascular system transports oxygen needed for cellular metabolism to the body's tissues and removes the carbon dioxide waste and brings it to the lungs. *Red blood cells* transport oxygen via *hemoglobin*, an iron-protein molecule. Hemoglobin also controls the rate of chemical reactions in cells by regulating hydrogen ion concentration. Strength and conditioning professionals should be aware that

blood doping, banned by most sport organizations, is the practice of artificially increasing the number of red blood cells to increase maximal oxygen uptake and enhance athletic performance. The practice can have serious health risks for athletes.

Respiratory System
Respiratory System Function
The respiratory system exchanges oxygen and carbon dioxide. Air first passes through the *nasal cavity* where it is purified, warmed, and humidified. Inspired air circulates to the lungs by going through the *trachea* (first-generation respiratory passage), the *right and left bronchi* (second-generation passages), and the *bronchioles* (third-generation passage). The bronchioles continue to divide for approximately twenty-three generations, down to the very small *alveoli,* where gas exchange during respiration occurs.

Exchange of Air and Respiratory Gases
The movement of air and expired gases, controlled by the expansion and recoil of the lungs, results from the *diaphragm* moving upward and downward (shortening and lengthening the chest cavity) and the movement of the ribs, which increases the anterior to posterior diameter of the chest cavity. During relaxed breathing, the contraction of the diaphragm during *inspiration* creates a negative pressure vacuum, drawing air into the lungs. The relaxation of the diaphragm causes an elastic recoil of the lungs, and the chest wall compresses the lungs, causing the air to be expelled. Heavy breathing during exercise requires extra force, provided by the contraction of the intercostals and muscles of the core, which push the abdomen upward against the diaphragm. Additionally, heavy breathing requires movement of the ribs to allow for expansion of the lungs. The ribs are elevated by muscles (external intercostals, sternocleidomastoids, anterior serrati, scaleni) during inspiration, allowing for more air to be inspired. The abdominal muscles and internal intercostals depress the chest during *expiration*. Expiration during resting conditions is passive but requires muscular contraction during exercise.

The walls of the lungs are composed of several layers of membranes, called *pleura*. *Pleural pressure* refers to the slightly negative pressure in the small spaces between the chest wall and lung pleura that enhances inspiration. Pleural pressure that is equal to or higher than atmospheric pressure will cause the lungs to collapse in a dangerous condition called a *pneumothorax*. When the glottis is open, no air moves in or out of the lungs, and the pressure inside the alveoli is referred to as *alveolar pressure*. Alveolar pressure must be below atmospheric pressure for inspiration to occur, and expiration requires an alveolar pressure higher than atmospheric pressure. The exchange of respiratory gases occurs when oxygen diffuses from the alveoli into pulmonary blood and carbon dioxide diffuses from blood into the alveoli. *Diffusion* of oxygen and carbon dioxide across cell membranes works according to a concentration gradient, where gas molecules move from regions of higher gas concentrations to regions of lower concentration. Note that the *Valsalva maneuver* results from abdominal muscle contraction with the diaphragm when the glottis is closed, causing an increase in intra-abdominal pressure during heavy weightlifting. This is thought to help stabilize the core and spine. Athletes should be aware that when the muscle contraction is too forceful, it can cause a hernia.

Cardiopulmonary Responses to Anaerobic and Aerobic Exercise

Anaerobic Exercise
Cardiovascular System
Acute anaerobic exercise causes increased cardiac output, heart rate, stroke volume, oxygen uptake, and systolic BP. Blood flow to active muscles also increases when lower resistances are used; however, decreased blood flow, resulting from the contracted muscle clamping down on capillaries, is observed with heavier resistance training. Muscular contractions greater than 20 percent of maximum voluntary

contraction slow peripheral blood flow during a set, but during rest, blood flow increases over that of baseline in a process called reactive hyperemia. Chronic resistance exercise can reduce the cardiovascular response to an acute bout of resistance exercise.

Respiratory System

Ventilation significantly increases during each resistance exercise set; however, ventilation is greatest during the first minute of recovery from a set. This increase in oxygen consumption via increased ventilation is termed excess post-oxygen consumption (EPOC). EPOC serves to help the body return to baseline after the work is performed and helps perfuse tissues to carry nutrients and remove waste, resynthesize hormones and metabolic intermediates, buffer lactate, etc.

Anaerobic training adaptations include increased tidal volume and breathing frequency with maximal resistance exercise, allowing for greater oxygen intake. Slower ventilation rates with increased tidal volume is seen with submaximal exercise.

Acute Aerobic Exercise

Cardiovascular System

Numerous cardiovascular responses occur in response to an acute bout of aerobic exercise including increased *cardiac output* (amount of blood pumped by the heart in liters/minute), *stroke volume* (quantity of blood ejected with each heart beat), heart rate, systolic BP, *oxygen uptake* (amount of oxygen used by the body's tissues), blood flow to working muscles, and *vasodilation* of blood vessels. Diastolic BP remains at resting levels or decreases slightly.

Respiratory System

Acute exercise results in a number of respiratory responses including increased amounts of oxygen diffusing to muscle tissue from the capillaries, increased tidal volume (amount of air inhaled and exhaled with each breath), increased movement of carbon dioxide diffusing from the blood into alveoli, as well as increased *minute ventilation (i.e., the volume of air breathed per minute)*, allowing the maintenance of appropriate alveolar concentrations of oxygen and carbon dioxide during acute aerobic activity. Excess *post-exercise oxygen consumption* may occur after an intense bout of exercise. Resting oxygen consumption is estimated to be 3.5 milliliters of oxygen per kilogram of body weight per minute; this value is defined as *1 metabolic equivalent (MET)*. An intense exercise bout can cause an increased metabolic demand that lasts for 6-12 hours after exercise.

Chronic Aerobic Exercise

Cardiovascular System

Aerobic endurance training produces several changes to cardiovascular functions that are critical for increasing maximal oxygen uptake and optimizing athletic performance. Aerobic endurance training increases cardiac output while decreasing resting heart rate. The normal discharge rate (60-80 times per minute) of the SA node slows significantly (due to increased parasympathetic tone), decreasing heart rate. At the same time, the increased stroke volume allows more blood to be pumped per contraction, so the heart can beat less frequently and still maintain the same cardiac output. Aerobic training can improve the ability of the heart to pump blood at rest, resulting in bradycardia in many highly-trained endurance athletes. An increase in maximal cardiac output is also observed, due to the increased stroke volume. Increased muscle fiber capillary density, enhancing the circulation of oxygen and nutrients and the removal of by-products, has been associated with aerobic endurance training. An athlete's genetic potential can significantly impact training adaptions. Aerobic capacity decreases with age, and men typically have greater aerobic capacity than women.

Respiratory System

Ventilation adaptations to aerobic endurance training are highly specific to the activity used in the training. If training focuses on the lower extremities (e.g., running), adaptations would not be observed during upper extremity exercise (e.g., arm ergometer exercise). Adaptations include increased tidal volume and breathing frequency during maximal exercise.

Adaptations to Metabolic Conditioning

Physiological adaptations to metabolic training are dependent upon the system stressed. High-intensity anaerobic training stresses the phosphagen system, resulting in physiological changes such as increased muscle strength, speed, rate of force production, and anaerobic power. Stressing the phosphagen system also results in increased metabolic stores of ATP, CP, and glycogen. Increases in the strength of connective tissue may be observed, while increases in various characteristics of muscle fibers (e.g., fiber cross-sectional area, myofibrillar volume, cytoplasmic density, myosin heavy chain protein) also occur.

Physiological adaptations to aerobic training include increases in cardiovascular and muscular endurance, mitochondrial and capillary density, ventricular size and strength, and metabolic stores of glycogen, adenosine triphosphate (ATP), and triglycerides. Highly-trained endurance athletes are also better equipped for glycogen sparing, wherein fat can provide fuel at higher intensities, allowing glycogen stores to be rationed to avoid "hitting the wall" as early. Increases in tendon and ligament strength and potentially in bone density also result from chronic high-impact cardiovascular activities.

Causes, Signs, Symptoms, and Effects of Overtraining and Detraining

Overtraining

Training overload (increased training intensity, volume, or duration) is required to stimulate the physiological adaptations that contribute to improved athletic performance; however, excessive overload combined with inadequate recovery can produce physiological maladaptation and diminished athletic performance. Training overload can lead to functional overreaching, nonfunctional overreaching, and overtraining syndrome (OTS). Training overload can lead to acute fatigue with recovery requiring days. Functional overreaching requires days to weeks of recovery, recovery from nonfunctional overreaching takes weeks to months, and OTS recovery requires months or longer. In some instances, OTS may end an athlete's sports career.

Overtraining Syndrome (OTS)

If training volume and/or intensity are increased and the athlete is unable to adequately recover and adapt, he or she may experience significant overload, resulting in OTS. Other variables experienced by athletes can also contribute to OTS, such as stress, lack of sleep, environmental variables (e.g., extreme heat, increasing the possibility of dehydration), and poor diet. There are two types of OTS: *sympathetic OTS* and *parasympathetic OTS*. It is believed that the sympathetic syndrome develops before parasympathetic syndrome. Sympathetic OTS is characterized by increased sympathetic activity at rest and is seen in young athletes in speed and power sports. Parasympathetic OTS is generally associated with aerobic overtraining and is characterized by increased parasympathetic activity at rest and during exercise.

Anaerobic (Sympathetic) OTS

Anaerobic (sympathetic) OTS is characterized by an unexplained decline in athletic performance that is associated with increased neural activity, mood disturbances (e.g., more tension, depression, fatigue), reduced immunity (e.g., resulting in increased sickness and infection), decreased skeletal muscle force

(F_M) production, reduced glycolytic capacity and appetite loss, and blunted increases in pituitary hormones such as ACTH and growth hormone.

<u>Aerobic (Parasympathetic) OTS</u>
Aerobic (parasympathetic) OTS is also characterized by poor athletic performance, including reduced performance on psychomotor tests. Other changes include reduced availability of glycogen, increased skeletal muscle soreness, increased levels of cortisol, decreased total testosterone concentration, mood changes, a greater sympathetic stress response, and reduced levels of nocturnal and resting catecholamines. Metabolism is affected by increased levels of creatine kinase and decreased lactate and cardiovascular alterations, including reduced oxygen uptake, increased resting heart rate, reduced heart rate variability, and altered BP. Some athletes experience weight gain and difficulty sleeping.

<u>Detraining</u>
If exercise volume and intensity decrease, the athlete will begin to lose the physiological adaptations achieved from training. Aerobic adaptations are most sensitive to inactivity. VO_2 max can be reduced by 4-14 percent after 4 weeks of reduced training stimulus and 6-20 percent after more than 4 weeks. Research has found that reduced maximal oxygen uptake results from several factors including decreased blood and stroke volume, reduced maximal cardiac output, and increased submaximal heart rate at a given workload.

Anatomical, Physiological, and Biomechanical Differences of Athletes

Several age-related terms will be used throughout this section. *Childhood* refers to the period of time prior to the development of secondary sex characteristics, while *adolescence* is the period between adulthood and childhood. *Youth* refers to both adolescents and children, and *older/elder/senior* refers to men and women who are over 65 years of age.

<u>Youth</u>
Growth, Development, and Maturation
Growth is an increase in the size of a body part or the entire body and results from an increase in the number of cells, while *development* refers to the progression that occurs from fetus to adult. *Maturation* is the process of the body becoming fully functional, which occurs at *puberty* when secondary sex characteristics develop, and the child transitions to adolescence. Note that changes that occur with puberty impact the individual's physical and motor skills, as well as body composition, and must be considered when developing training programs.

Chronological, Biological, and Training Age
There is substantial variation in the growth and development rates of children, so age can be understood from three perspectives. *Chronological age* refers to the years and months the child has been alive. Children of the same chronological age can be at different stages of development and maturation. To take pubertal development (e.g., skeletal age, somatic [body shape] sexual maturation) into consideration, *biological age* can be used. Children having the same chronological age but different biological ages have varying levels of motor skills, muscular strength, and fitness. Biological age should be used when grouping children for fitness testing and athletic competitions, providing fairer matching of physical and athletic abilities. The gold standard method of determining biological age is to assess skeletal age via x-rays or radiographs of the wrist or iliac crest to compare bone ossification to standard reference radiographs. One additional factor that should be considered when developing a youth training program is *training age*, which is the length of time the youth has been doing a formal, supervised resistance training program.

Youth Resistance Training Program
When developing a resistance program for youth, strength and conditioning professionals must be mindful that the youth athlete is *not* a miniature adult. It is important that youth begin resistance training programs based on their previous training experience, maturity level, physical abilities, and goals; it is always better to underestimate ability level and gradually increase volume and intensity. Research has demonstrated that preadolescent girls and boys can significantly improve their muscular strength beyond the natural improvement associated with growth and maturation. Changes in muscle hypertrophy may be partially responsible for increased strength, but increased strength is primarily due to neurological factors such as motor unit recruitment, activation, synchronization, and firing. The two most important factors in the development of a youth program are the quality of instruction such as the demonstration of appropriate technique and employing the appropriate rate of progression. In general, the program should include various single- and multi-joint resistance exercises with sets of six to fifteen repetitions using light resistance with two to three nonconsecutive sessions per week. For younger children, body weight usually provides sufficient resistance, and the use of resistance bands can augment training stimulus, where appropriate. It is important to focus on basic movement patterns involving large-muscle groups (squats, lunges, dead lifts, push-ups), emphasizing proper form and breathing to help develop foundational strength training patterns and to prevent injuries.

Older Adults
Many changes in body composition and neuromotor function are observed among adults over the age of sixty-five. Bones become fragile with age because of reduced bone mineral density (BMD), increasing the risk for fractures, particularly of the spine, hip, and wrist. *Osteopenia* refers to a BMD level that is between -1 and -2.5 standard deviations of the BMD of young adults, and *osteoporosis* is a BMD of 2.5 standard deviations below that of young adults. *Sarcopenia* is the loss of muscle mass, and therefore, strength and power. It is largely due to reduced levels of physical activity but can also be impacted by poor nutrition and hormonal and nervous system changes. Neuromotor functional changes can lead to increased risk of falling (and fractures due to reduced BMD) and can result from decreased strength and power, longer reaction time, and impairments in balance and postural stability. Older adults use strategies such as increased muscle activity before *(preactivation)* and immediately following *(cocontraction)* contact with the ground. Increased muscle tension associated with preactivation and the joint stabilization provided by cocontraction can help to offset balance and postural problems. Multidimensional programs that consist of resistance and balance exercises result in the most improvement of neuromotor function in seniors. Aging does not decrease the body's ability to adapt to resistance exercise, so it is possible to see large improvements in muscle mass, power, strength, BMD, and motor function (e.g., walking speed). Although both aerobic and balance exercises are important and should be included in a training program, resistance training is needed to increase muscle strength, power, and mass. Resistance training programs for older adults are similar to programs for younger adults; however, medical history, training history, nutrition, and other variables should be considered. All older adults should complete a *medical history* with a *risk factor questionnaire* prior to beginning a training program. The safety recommendations for resistance training in older adults are similar to many of those for other age groups (e.g., 5-10 minutes of warm-up, stretching after exercise, allowing 48-72 hours between training sessions).

Female Athletes
Women can gain many benefits from regular participation in resistance and aerobic exercise. It is important for strength and conditioning professionals to understand sex-related differences in body composition, strength, and physiological responses to resistance exercise to design an appropriate resistance program that will optimize athletic performance without increasing the risk of sport-related

injuries. When females reach puberty, estrogen production increases fat deposition. On average, adult females weigh less than males but have a higher percentage of body fat and less lean mass. When considering absolute strength, females have about two-thirds the strength of males, with lower body strength being closer to that of males as compared to upper body strength. When strength is related to body weight, females have similar levels of lower body strength as males; however, the relative upper body strength of females is still less than that of males. Importantly, when strength is expressed relative to the cross-sectional area of a muscle, no strength differences exist between males and females, indicating that muscle quality is not sex-specific. Women and men respond similarly to resistance training. Two important health risks specific to women are the *female athlete triad* and the increased risk (i.e., six times greater risk among females than males) of *anterior cruciate ligament (ACL) tears* of the knee. The female triad refers to the interrelationships between BMD, energy availability, and menstrual function. Females participating in heavy training volumes and/or intensities with insufficient caloric intake are at risk for osteoporosis and *amenorrhea* (i.e., the absence of a menstrual cycle for more than 3 months), and these increase the risk of stress fractures, endocrine and reproductive problems, and performance decrements. Training programs for females and males can be similar, the only difference being the amount of resistance used. Women participating in sports requiring upper body strength and those that put the knee at risk for injury can benefit from resistance exercises to strengthen these areas.

Psychological Techniques Used to Enhance Training and Performance

Ideal Performance State
Often referred to as "the zone," athletes report the ideal performance state is characterized by several components including 1) a sense of personal control, 2) a feeling of effortless performance, 3) an absence of a fear of failure, 4) attention focused on the activity being performed, 5) performing the activity without having to think about or analyze it, and 6) a feeling that time slows. down

Motivational Techniques
Motivation, a psychological construct, is the direction and intensity of an athlete's effort. There are several forms of motivation including intrinsic and extrinsic motivation, achievement motivation, and motivation associated with skill development. It should be noted that athletes generally experience more than one type of motivation, and these can vary depending on the activity being performed, perceptions of competency, the level of importance the athlete places on the activity, and other factors.

Intrinsic Motivation
Intrinsic motivation is an athlete's internal desire for his or her behavior to be competent and self-determined. It originates from the athlete's love and interest in the sport and personal satisfaction (inherent reward) in performing the activity. Intrinsic motivation is generally considered the best form of motivation. It can help an athlete maintain focus on achieving short-term goals that require consistent effort to enhance the athlete's performance level.

Extrinsic Motivation
Extrinsic motivation, used extensively in sports, comes from external sources (e.g., coaches, teammates) in the form of individualized rewards such as praise from coaches and teammates, medals, social acceptance, avoidance of punishment, and the desire for positive reinforcement.

Achievement Motivation
Achievement motivation reflects an athlete's effort to master a specific task, achieve excellence, perform better than others, and overcome obstacles. Athletes with high levels of achievement

motivation are more competitive and generally perform better than athletes with lower levels of achievement motivation. There are two types of achievement motivation. The motive to achieve success (MAS) is characterized by a desire to challenge and evaluate one's ability and be proud of accomplishments. Athletes with greater MAS like challenging situations, where the likelihood of success or failure is approximately the same. The motive to avoid failure (MAF) is characterized by the desire to avoid being perceived as a failure, preserve one's ego and self-confidence, and minimize shame. Athletes with greater MAF prefer either easy situations where they will likely succeed and avoid shame or difficult situations where success is unlikely and feelings of shame are minimized.

Reinforcement Strategies

Positive Reinforcement

The goal of positive reinforcement is to increase the occurrence of a favorable behavior (e.g., skill, movement, appropriate teamwork) or outcome (e.g., improved performance). Immediately after the positive behavior occurs, the athlete or team is given a positive incentive. This incentive is something that the athlete/team values (praise, more playing time, starting position, extra rest between sets, etc.) to encourage continued occurrence of the desired positive behavior.

Negative Reinforcement

Similar to positive reinforcement, negative reinforcement provides a "reward" after the occurrence of the desired behavior or outcome. This reward is the removal of a stimulus the athlete/team views as aversive. A strength and conditioning coach might remove the regularly performed sets of push-ups after the entire team performed an exercise using the correct technique.

Positive Punishment

Positive punishment is used to deter undesirable behavior by presenting an action, object, or event after the unwanted behavior occurs. Positive punishment might take the form of an athlete running extra sprints after practice because he or she was late or a team receiving a reprimand from the coach after incorrectly running a specific play.

Negative Punishment

Negative punishment involves the removal of a highly valued positive stimulus after an unwanted behavior or outcome occurs to deter future occurrences of the behavior. A team that is joking around during a resistance training session may receive negative punishment when the strength and conditioning coach turns off the music for the remainder of the training session.

Imagery Techniques

Imagery techniques utilize mental visualization of specific athletic situations such as the performance of a targeted event/race. The benefits of vivid imagery include providing an athlete with exposure to the successful execution of a specific skill under a stressful competitive situation (e.g., sinking a putt on the eighteenth hole); allowing the athlete to "experience" the sights, sounds, smells, and physical exertion associated with the competitive environment on a regular basis and at a much greater frequency than actual competitions during the season; and the athlete feeling (or watching) himself or herself perform successfully and gaining confidence in the ability to perform optimally.

Methods that Enhance Motor Learning and Skill Acquisition

Instruction

There are three main types of instruction that can be used with athletes: explicit instruction, guided discovery, and discovery. *Explicit instruction* facilitates the athlete's learning by providing the most information about the task in a prescriptive manner, aimed at guiding the athlete through the entire movement, often in a step-by-step fashion. *Guided discovery* gives less information to the athlete than explicit instruction but provides a more holistic description of the overall movement. By providing the goal of the task and some details about the movement, the athlete has to integrate the information provided with the movement pattern being practiced to understand how the goal is related to the movements performed. *Discovery* provides no instructions, but rather presents the overall goal of a movement. Using discovery-oriented instruction gives the athlete an opportunity to explore various methods to achieve the movement goal; however, it can be time-intensive.

Feedback
Feedback plays a critical role in the acquisition and refinement of new motor skills. In general, when learning a new movement skill, it is beneficial to provide more frequent feedback that decreases over time as mastery is reached. The athlete has readily accessible *intrinsic feedback* provided by his or her body and sensory systems. An athlete kicks a soccer ball, and sensory information from the athlete's eyes, proprioceptors, mechanoreceptors, and joint receptors in the foot provides intrinsic feedback that the he or she can utilize to refine the movement. *Augmented feedback* originates from an external source, such as a coach, other observer, or technology (e.g., video, heart rate monitor, laboratory equipment). Two types of augmented feedback are *knowledge of results* and *knowledge of performance*. The difference between these two forms of feedback is whether information provided to the athlete is about the completion of a movement task (i.e., the amount of time the task took) or the athlete's performance of the movement task (e.g., the position of the athlete's feet).

Whole vs. Part Practice
When learning a complex motor skill, there are two different strategies: whole vs. part practice. *Whole practice* is required with complex motor skills because the component movements are interrelated (such as in archery or performing a jump shot). It also works well for skills that are not particularly complex. *Part practice* is best used to teach athletes complex skills with subcomponents that are less interrelated, such as a gymnastics floor routine.

Attentional Control and Decision-Making Skills

Arousal
In sports, arousal is the intensity of motivation, anxiety, and focus experienced by an athlete and is the result of physiological and psychological activation. Arousal can be understood as a continuum of activation from deep sleep to very intense excitement. A highly-aroused athlete may experience an increased heart rate, sweating, and anxiety, while the athlete with low arousal may be lying down and feel tired and unfocused. Optimal arousal is often described as an inverse "U," wherein the ideal performance occurs with moderate levels of arousal, while either extreme can detract from performance. Arousal can be associated with both pleasant and unpleasant situations and interpreted as being a positive or negative to an athlete.

Anxiety
Anxiety is perceived as a negative emotional state, associated with the body being physiologically aroused, which is generally characterized by worry, nervousness, apprehension, and fear. The thought process responsible for the perception of anxiety as negative is a result of *cognitive anxiety*, while its counterpart, *somatic anxiety*, is the physical symptoms (e.g., increased heart rate, upset stomach) of anxiety. Previous negative outcomes (e.g., false start on a relay) and negative thoughts may manifest physically, negatively impacting the physical performance of the athlete. Recognizing how negative physical and psychological arousal impacts an athlete's mental state and performance can provide an opportunity to assist the athlete in understanding his or her reaction to anxiety in stressful situations.

The athlete can begin working on perceiving the stressful situations more positively and to control the anxiety.

Additionally, anxiety can also be categorized as trait or state anxiety. *Trait anxiety* is considered to be part of one's personality, predisposing an athlete to perceive many situations as being threatening when in fact, no physical or psychological danger exists. In general, athletes with high trait anxiety generally experience higher levels of state anxiety. *State anxiety* is a continually changing component of mood that is the subjective perception of tension and apprehension associated with increased arousal of the autonomic and endocrine systems. An athlete's level of state anxiety may change throughout a soccer game with changing situations and may have a positive, negative, or no impact on performance, depending upon the athlete's skill level, difficulty of tasks being performed, and his or her level of trait anxiety.

Stress
Stress is the result of a psychological and/or physical demand placed on an athlete who does not have the ability to respond to the demand. The situation causing this imbalance of demand and response – an environmental or cognitive stressor – causes a stress response. Stress can be positive *(eustress)* or negative *(distress)* for an athlete. Training places a physiological stress on the body that is required for an athlete to improve performance.

Influence of Arousal and Anxiety on Performance

Drive Theory
Drive theory considers the relationship between arousal and performance to be linear; the more arousal experienced by the athlete, the better the he or she will perform. Clearly, this is not the case, as too much or too little arousal can negatively impact performance. Two factors that significantly impact how an athlete's level of arousal influences performance are *skill level* and *task complexity*. Athletes at lower skill levels need less arousal to perform than their highly skilled counterparts because less skilled or new athletes must concentrate on the actions being performed; too many apprehensive thoughts can interfere with the unskilled athlete's ability to concentrate. Lower levels of arousal are also advantageous for athletes attempting difficult tasks that require a lot of conscious attention. For example, hockey goalies perform better with lower levels of arousal than athletes whose tasks do not require an extensive amount of attention. In contrast, long-distant runners can perform well at a higher level of arousal because the biomechanical task (running, in this case) is somewhat automatic and does not require a significant amount of conscious attention.

Arousal Management

Inverted-U Theory
As mentioned, the inverted-U theory posits that too little or too much arousal negatively impacts athletic performance, and there is an optimal level of arousal that facilitates optimal performance. The inverted-U graphically shows this (x-axis is level of arousal; y-axis is performance), as the shape demonstrates that low levels or high levels beyond the optimal level of arousal result in worse performance, and somewhere between low and high arousal is the range of arousal associated with optimal performance (the top of the inverted-U). At this point, the internal and external stimuli experienced by the athlete generate the optimal amount of arousal required to enhance performance. For example, if the heart rate is not fast enough, the body might not be physiologically ready to perform, but a heart rate that is too fast can cause fatigue too early in the competition, negatively impacting

performance. As mentioned, athletes vary greatly in the level of arousal needed for optimal performance depending on a variety of factors.

Individual Zones of Optimal Functioning (IZOF) Theory

This theory recognizes that there is a continuum of state anxiety that varies across athletes and that emotions can also impact an athlete's optimal zone of functioning. It is the role of the coach to help the athletes identify and reach their optimal level of state anxiety. This can be accomplished by quantifying state anxiety and mood using specific assessments. By quantifying state anxiety, it is possible to identify each athlete's ideal range of state anxiety needed to enhance performance and optimize the athlete's abilities.

Catastrophe Theory

Catastrophe theory recognizes that cognitive and somatic anxiety, along with physiological arousal, can negatively impact optimal arousal levels, leading to an abrupt decline in athletic performance. Cognitive anxiety taking effect after the arousal threshold has been reached can quickly and detrimentally impact an athlete's thought process, causing the athlete to focus on and doubt his or her ability to perform, resulting in a devastating performance decline.

Reversal Theory

Reversal theory simply states that high levels of arousal and anxiety experienced by an athlete can be perceived positively as an indication that the athlete is excited and ready to compete, or negatively as unpleasant, as demonstrated by a lack confidence. For the athlete to perform optimally, arousal must be interpreted positively. This theory is novel because 1) the athlete's interpretation of the arousal—not the amount felt—is important, and 2) the athlete has the ability to change negative interpretations of arousal into positive interpretations, thus controlling the response to high levels of arousal.

Relaxation Techniques

Diaphragmatic Breathing

Diaphragmatic breathing is a technique that can easily be taught and used by athletes to aid physical and mental relaxation. It distracts the mind from focusing on stress because it requires attention on the mechanics of breathing and the abdominal region. This technique can help reduce heart rate and muscle tension, decrease autonomic nervous system functioning, and increase parasympathetic nervous system activity, resulting in deep relaxation due to the reduced neural stimulation of the muscles and organs.

Progressive Muscular Relaxation

Progressive muscular relaxation can be used by athletes to control pre-competition levels of somatic and cognitive activation to regulate levels of physical and psychological arousal. It essentially consists of contracting and relaxing muscle groups until the entire body is relaxed. This form of relaxation increases the athlete's awareness of somatic tension, with the hope that relaxing the body will result in a relaxed mind.

Autogenic Training

Autogenic training is a series of exercises using a type of self-hypnosis that are aimed at increasing the sensations of warmth and heaviness in various body parts. The athlete gets in a comfortable position and then focuses on five stages of relaxation that move from a focus on the heaviness and then warmth of the extremities, the regulation of cardiac activity and breathing, abdominal warmth, and finally, cooling of the forehead.

Systematic Desensitization (fear)

This technique utilizes a skill-based relaxation response to control cognitive arousal. In a controlled environment, the athlete visualizes the particular experience that causes fear (e.g., diver hit his head on the board during competition) while simultaneously using breathing and muscle relaxation techniques. Progressive imagery helps that athlete to visualize the entire fear-causing experience without trying to cognitively avoid the situation. This counterconditioning replaces the fear response with relaxation.

Attention and Focus

Attention and Selective Attention

Attention refers to an athlete's awareness of internal and environmental cues. Athletes in a competitive or training environment face a continual barrage of external stimuli and internal thoughts, some of which are important for performance. *Selective attention* is one's ability to focus on relevant, task-oriented cues while ignoring other stimuli and thoughts irrelevant to the athletic performance at hand. The soccer player needs to stay focused on the location of the players of both teams while ignoring cheering from the crowds or announcements being made at the adjacent field. Those athletes capable of focusing on task-relevant sensory input will experience a higher level of performance in comparison to the athlete who finds it difficult to block out input that is not task-related.

Confidence and Positive Self-Talk and Goal Setting

Self-Confidence

Self-confidence is the belief in one's ability to perform a specific behavior such as hitting a baseball or completing a marathon. In the realm of sports, research has identified several types of self-confidence including self-confidence in performing physical skills, in one's ability to use psychological skills (e.g., self-talk) and perceptual skills (e.g., visual scanning), one's learning potential (needed to improve skills), and confidence in one's training and level of fitness.

Self-Efficacy

Self-efficacy (SE) is the athlete's perception of his or her ability to perform a situation-specific task successfully. The strength and conditioning professional should recognize that his or her actions can improve the athlete's SE by targeting the multiple sources that influence SE. The first and most significant source of SE is the athlete's past performance experiences. Helping the athlete set challenging but attainable short-term goals can provide performance success, which can have a positive impact on SE. The second source is vicarious experiences where the athlete watches/models a similar athlete's successful performance (e.g., "If someone similar to me can complete that new drill, so can I."). Verbal persuasion, the third SE source, can include encouragement from coaches, teammates, oneself, and other external sources (e.g., Nike's "Just Do It" slogan). The fourth source of SE is physiological arousal and emotional/mood states. For example, helping an athlete interpret pre-competition "jitteriness" as excitement to compete because the athlete knows he or she can successfully achieve a specific performance goal can positively influence SE, as opposed to the interpretation of the "jitteriness" as a sign of being nervous or unprepared to compete.

Self-Talk

Positive self-talk provides motivation ("I can get my personal best time in this race!"), encouragement ("Get ready to swim fast!"), and reinforcement ("I am prepared for this race!") and often is used to increase effort, energy, and a positive attitude. When an athlete uses *instructional self-talk*, he or she generally focuses on technical and task-related aspects of performance ("Streamline off the wall!") or strategy ("Maintain my race pace for this 800-meter run."). *Negative self-talk* typically denotes anger

("Can't believe I missed that putt. I'm such an idiot and will never win now."), doubt ("I can't do this."), negative judgment ("That was not good enough."), or discouragement ("There is no way I can win this race.").

Goal Setting

Effective goal setting requires a systematic approach to ensure the goals positively impact both the physical and psychological development of the athlete. For goal setting to be successful, goals need to be specific, challenging but attainable, and outcome- and process-oriented, and include interdependent short- and long-term goals.

Process Goals

Process goals are focused on the actions that are required to execute a skill or perform well. Focusing on the actions rather than the final result increases the athlete's control over achieving the desired results. Obtaining a process goal is dependent on expenditure of effort by the athlete to alter his or her actions.

Outcome Goals

Outcome goals usually focus on a result of a competitive event, such as setting a world record. Obtaining these goals is not under the athlete's control because these outcomes are dependent on the effort and performance of both the athlete and others. Using process goals to achieve outcome goals can facilitate the development of obtainable daily goals. This can help to lessen the focus on the end result and help the athlete maintain the motivation and effort required to reach the final result.

Short- and Long-Term Goals

A staircase is a useful metaphor for understanding short- and long-term goals. Each individual step is a short-term goal, and the top of the staircase is the long-term goal. The athlete's current ability level is the bottom step, and each step moving toward the top is a series of progressively more challenging short-term process-oriented goals that are linked to the top step, representing the long-term outcome goal.

Practice Questions

1. Which of the following is NOT a component of a sarcomere?
    a. Actin
    b. D-line
    c. A-band
    d. I-band

2. Which of the following best describes the likely ratio of Type I and Type II muscle fibers in a competitive tennis player?
    a. High Type I, low Type II
    b. High Type I, high Type II
    c. Low Type I, high Type II
    d. Low Type I, low Type II

3. Which of the following correctly lists the structures of a muscle from largest to smallest?
    a. Fasciculus, muscle fiber, actin, myofibril
    b. Muscle fiber, fasciculus, myofibril, actin
    c. Sarcomere, fasciculus, myofibril, myosin
    d. Muscle fiber, myofibril, sarcomere, actin

4. What area of the heart is responsible for initiating rhythmic electrical impulses?
    a. Purkinje fibers
    b. Atrioventricular (AV) bundle
    c. Sinoatrial (SA) node
    d. Atrioventricular (AV) node

5. When reading an electrocardiogram, ventricular repolarization is associated with which graphical component?
    a. QRS complex
    b. P-wave
    c. T-wave
    d. PR segment

6. Which of the following are responsible for the exchange of nutrients, hormones, oxygen, fluids, and electrolytes between blood and the interstitial fluid of body tissues?
    a. Arterioles
    b. Venules
    c. Capillaries
    d. Hemoglobin

7. Myosin cross-bridges attach to the actin filament when the sarcoplasmic reticulum is stimulated to release which one of the following?
    a. Calcium ions
    b. Acetylcholine
    c. Troponin
    d. Adenosine triphosphate (ATP)

8. During heavy breathing, which of the following muscles do NOT help to elevate the ribs during inspiration?
   a. Sternocleidomastoids
   b. External intercostals
   c. Rectus abdominis
   d. Anterior serrati

9. Which of the following sport-related movements occurs primarily in the transverse plane?
   a. Dribbling a soccer ball
   b. Hitting a tennis backhand
   c. Punting a football
   d. Throwing a shot put

10. Which of the following muscles does NOT rotate the arm?
    a. Teres minor
    b. Subscapularis
    c. Infraspinatus
    d. Supinator

11. A biceps curl is an example of which type of lever?
    a. First-class lever
    b. Second-class lever
    c. Third-class lever
    d. Fourth-class lever

12. Which of the following upper body movements take place in the sagittal plane?
    I. Elbow extension
    II. Wrist flexion
    III. Shoulder abduction
    IV. Neck left tilt

    a. I, IV
    b. I, III, IV
    c. I, II
    d. II, III

13. Soccer dribbling requires what joint movement at the ankle and in which movement plane?
    a. Eversion/transverse
    b. Inversion/frontal
    c. Eversion/frontal
    d. Inversion/transverse

14. Which one of the following answers provides the correct name and fascicular arrangement description associated with the biceps brachii muscle?
    a. Fusiform; spindle-shaped muscles
    b. Multipennate; tendon branches within the muscle
    c. Longitudinal (AKA: parallel); long axis of fascicles are parallel to long axis of muscle
    d. Radiate (AKA: convergent); muscle has broad origin (fan or triangular shape)

15. Which of the following refers to when a muscle contracts but does not shorten or lengthen?
    a. Eccentric
    b. Isotonic
    c. Concentric
    d. Isometric

16. Which of the following is the equation for power?
    a. Force × distance
    b. Work/time
    c. Work/distance
    d. Force × time

17. A collegiate track sprinter is doing interval training at a 1:12 work-to-rest ratio. This type of training is working what energy system?
    a. Fast glycolysis and oxidative
    b. Oxidative
    c. Fast glycolysis
    d. Phosphagen

18. Which substrate is capable of producing the most ATP?
    a. Carbohydrates
    b. Fat
    c. Protein
    d. Glycogen

19. The electron transport chain resynthesizes ATP by the process of oxidative phosphorylation. Which of the following is NOT used during this process?
    a. Hydrogen ions
    b. Lactate
    c. Nicotinamide adenine dinucleotide (NADH)
    d. Flavin adenine dinucleotide (FADH$_2$)

20. The phosphagen system uses creatine phosphate stored in muscles to produce ATP. Which of the following is NOT true about the reaction?
    a. The reaction produces energy at a fast rate.
    b. The reaction uses the process of substrate-level phosphorylation to resynthesize ATP.
    c. The reaction uses the process of oxidative phosphorylation to resynthesize ATP.
    d. The reaction is not capable of providing energy for continuous, long-duration activity.

21. Which of the energy systems is the primary system working when the body is at rest?
    a. Glycolysis
    b. Oxidative
    c. Anaerobic
    d. Phosphagen

22. What is the net production of ATP from the complete metabolism of one molecule of glucose?
    a. 4
    b. 24
    c. 38
    d. 40

23. The process of breaking large molecules into smaller molecules to provide energy is known as which of the following?
    a. Metabolism
    b. Bioenergetics
    c. Anabolism
    d. Catabolism

24. If oxygen is available during glycolysis, what happens to pyruvate?
    a. It is converted to lactate.
    b. It is transported to the sarcoplasm for the Krebs cycle.
    c. It is transported to the mitochondria for the Krebs cycle.
    d. It is converted to lactic acid.

25. Cortisol is secreted by which of the following?
    a. Adrenal cortex
    b. Anterior pituitary
    c. Posterior pituitary
    d. Testes and ovaries

26. Which of the following is NOT an anabolic hormone?
    a. Testosterone
    b. Growth hormone
    c. Insulin-like growth factor
    d. Epinephrine

27. Which of the following is not a physiological function of testosterone?
    a. Increases protein synthesis
    b. Increases the rate of cellular metabolism
    c. Increases cardiac output
    d. Increases the production of red blood cells

28. What type of resistance exercise training promotes increased concentrations of growth hormone?

	Number of Sets	Intensity	Rest Interval
a.	3	High	1 minute
b.	3	Low	3 minutes
c.	1	High	1 minute
d.	1	Low	3 minutes

29. Which of the following is not a function of catecholamines?
    a. Decreases blood pressure
    b. Increases available energy
    c. Increases rate of muscle contraction
    d. Increases muscle blood flow

30. Which of the following resistance exercise variables would best enhance serum testosterone concentrations?
    a. Long rest intervals (greater than 2 minutes)
    b. Small-muscle exercises such as biceps curls
    c. Heavy resistance loads (85-95 percent of 1RM)
    d. One set of each resistance exercise

31. Endocrine signs and symptoms associated with overtraining syndrome include all EXCEPT which of the following?
    a. Altered cortisol concentrations
    b. Increased growth hormone
    c. Decreased total testosterone concentration
    d. Decreased ratios of total and free testosterone to cortisol

32. The following list of physiological functions are associated with which hormone? Physiological functions: decreases glucose utilization, increases protein synthesis, increases renal plasma flow and filtration, and enhances immune cell function.
    a. Insulin-like growth factor
    b. Testosterone
    c. Growth hormone
    d. Epinephrine

33. Which of the following characteristics of the mechanical load associated with resistance exercises are important for the stimulation of bone growth?
    I. Speed of the loading
    II. Intensity of the loading
    III. Direction of the force
    IV. Type of load
    a. I, III, IV
    b. II, III, IV
    c. I, II, III
    d. I, II, III, IV

34. High-intensity resistance training causes all muscle fibers to hypertrophy because of the order of motor unit recruitment. What is the name of this phenomenon where smaller motor units are recruited first, followed by the recruitment of larger units when more force is needed?
    a. Selective recruitment
    b. The size principle
    c. Maximal recruitment
    d. Synchronization of motor unit activation

35. High-intensity anaerobic training causes changes to connective tissue growth and structure. Which of the following is NOT a change that occurs in tendons in response to this training?
    a. Increased collagen fibril diameter and number
    b. Increased tendon flexibility
    c. Increased formation of long filaments
    d. Increased collagen fibril packing density

36. An acute bout of anaerobic resistance exercise significantly impacts the cardiovascular system. During resistance exercise, which cardiovascular responses occur?

    I. Increased heart rate and systolic blood pressure

    II. Increased cardiac output

    III. Increased peripheral blood flow

    IV. Increased stroke volume

  a. I, II

  b. I, II, III

  c. I, II, IV

  d. I, II, III, IV

37. At what point during acute resistance exercise sets is ventilation the greatest?

  a. Immediately before starting the resistance exercise set

  b. During the resistance exercise set

  c. During the first minute of recovery from the exercise set

  d. After the resistance exercise training session is completed

38. Increased tendon stiffness is associated with which of the following?

  a. Greater muscular recoil and power production

  b. Decreased ability of tendon to withstand tensional forces

  c. Enhanced muscular flexibility

  d. Increased risk of injury

39. Which of the following collegiate athletes is most likely to have low bone mineral density?

  a. A swimmer who runs during preseason and has two resistance training sessions per week during the season

  b. A lacrosse player who plays midfielder

  c. A gymnast whose primary events are the floor exercise and the vault

  d. A distance cyclist with one resistance training session per week

40. Which of the following is NOT true about the impact of aerobic training on bone growth?

  a. High-intensity activities such as running or aerobics are required to stimulate bone growth.

  b. The intensity of the activity must continue to increase systematically to ensure that the bones experience continual overload.

  c. Any type of high-intensity aerobic activity can stimulate bone growth.

  d. If the intensity of the activity cannot be increased, increasing the rate of the limb movement can continue to stimulate bone growth.

41. Which of the following is a common adaptation to aerobic endurance training that athletes can easily measure?

  a. Resting heart rate

  b. Stroke volume

  c. Systolic blood pressure

  d. Diastolic blood pressure

42. An aerobic endurance athlete experiencing detraining will first experience a decline in what?
 a. Maximal oxygen consumption
 b. Resting heart rate
 c. Stroke volume
 d. Muscular strength

43. Adaptations to aerobic endurance training include all but which of the following?
 a. Increased blood lactate concentrations
 b. Increased stroke volume
 c. Increased blood flow to working muscles
 d. increased cardiac output

44. Which of the following individual characteristics that influence adaptations to aerobic endurance training can be controlled by the athlete?
 a. Age
 b. Sex
 c. Negative health behaviors (e.g., smoking)
 d. Genetic potential

45. Which of the following is NOT a sign or symptom of aerobic overtraining syndrome?
 a. Increased resting heart rate
 b. Reduced oxygen uptake
 c. Increased muscle glycogen
 d. Increased cortisol concentration

46. A strength and conditioning professional is developing a resistance training program for a youth athlete who has 3 years of resistance training experience. Which age (based on the information that the age provides) would be the most important to consider while developing the training program?
 a. Biological age
 b. Training age
 c. Chronological age
 d. Skeletal age

47. Many factors go into the development of a resistance training program for youth. Which of the following components are necessary to create the best program possible for the athlete?
 I. Quality of instruction by the strength and conditioning professional
 II. Including an appropriate rate of progression
 III. Treating the athlete as a miniature adult
 IV. Scheduling training sessions as nonconsecutive sessions to allow appropriate recovery

 a. I, II
 b. II, III
 c. I, II, IV
 d. I, III, IV

48. Youth experience improvements in strength, agility, and power primarily because of the development of which system?
    a. The musculoskeletal system
    b. The nervous system
    c. The respiratory system
    d. The cardiovascular system

49. Which of the following is true about muscle strength in women?
    a. Women have about 1/2 the absolute body strength as compared to men.
    b. The absolute upper body strength of women is similar to men.
    c. When strength is related to body weight, females and males have similar lower body strength levels.
    d. When strength is expressed as cross-sectional area of a muscle, females have about 2/3 the strength of men.

50. Which of the following is NOT an aspect of the female athlete triad?
    a. Anterior cruciate ligament (ACL) tears
    b. Amenorrhea
    c. Energy availability
    d. Bone mineral density

51. A 69-year-old women would like to begin a resistance training program and knows that her physical inactivity has resulted in strength loss but does not know if it has impacted her bone mineral density. A bone density scan showed that her bone mineral density level was 1.5 standard deviations below the bone mineral density of young adults. Based on these results, what condition is the women experiencing?
    a. Reduced neuromotor functioning
    b. Osteopenia
    c. Sarcopenia
    d. Osteoporosis

52. Which of the following does not need to be considered when developing an optimal training program for an older adult?
    a. Medical history
    b. Risk factor questionnaire
    c. Resistance and aerobic training history
    d. The older adult's request for the program to contain only resistance exercises

53. Although Robert is not the best basketball player on the team, he loves participating in the game and having the opportunity to work on new skills. He also is good at maintaining his focus on achieving his short-term goals. What type of motivation is driving Robert's behavior?
    a. Extrinsic motivation
    b. Achievement motivation
    c. Outcome motivation
    d. Intrinsic motivation

54. The ideal performance state can be characterized by all BUT which of the following?
    a. The absence of fear
    b. A high level of arousal
    c. A sense of personal control
    d. A narrow focus of attention on the activity

55. A gymnast getting ready to perform her last routine in the all-around competition is worried about the routine and is experiencing an increased heart rate, sweating, and "butterflies." The physical symptoms experienced by the gymnast are associated with which type of anxiety?
    a. Environmental anxiety
    b. Physical anxiety
    c. Cognitive anxiety
    d. Somatic anxiety

56. Beth has elevated levels of psychological arousal prior to competing that have been detrimental to her performance. She recently learned a new relaxation technique that uses a series of alternating muscle tensing followed by a muscle relaxation phase. What specific technique is Beth using to reduce arousal?
    a. Diaphragmatic breathing
    b. Imagery
    c. Progressive muscular relaxation
    d. Systematic desensitization

57. A basketball player getting ready to shoot a free throw blocks out the opposing players and noisy crowd in order to focus on making the shot. This behavior is an example of which of the following?
    a. Internal attention
    b. Selective attention
    c. Focus
    d. Optimal functioning

58. A swimmer obtained her best time in the 100-yard butterfly during a split squad meet at the beginning of the training season. This is an example of what type of self-efficacy source?
    a. Vicarious experience
    b. Mastery performance accomplishment
    c. Verbal persuasion
    d. Physiological states

59. Sarah is learning how to do the long jump, an event that she never participated in during high school. Which type of motor skill learning may be best for her coach to implement for this event?
    a. Part practice
    b. Guided discovery
    c. Whole practice
    d. Discovery

60. John met with his coach to outline his goals for performing the 5000-meter race. One goal is to maintain his running form during the final 400 meters of the race. What type of goal is this?
    a. Short-term goal
    b. Outcome goal
    c. Long-term goal
    d. Process goal

Answer Explanations

1. B: Sarcomeres are the smallest functional unit of a muscle and contain the actin and myosin proteins responsible for the mechanical process of muscle contractions. Sarcomeres are divided into sections or regions based on the presence of the contractile proteins. The A-band, H-zone, I-band, and Z-line are defined regions within a sarcomere.

2. B: Tennis requires significant involvement of both Type I (slow-twitch) and Type II (fast-twitch) muscle fibers. Type I muscle fibers have a high capacity for aerobic energy supply and are fatigue-resistant—two traits that allow the player to maintain performance levels over multiple sets. Type II muscle fibers are easily fatigable but are capable of high force development, which is beneficial for short sprints to the ball, etc. Large locomotor muscles, such as the quadriceps, have a mixture of Type I and Type II fibers.

3. D: Muscle fibers or myocytes are long, striated, cylindrical cells that are approximately the diameter of a human hair (50-100 micrometers), are multinucleated, and are covered by a fibrous membrane called the sarcolemma, which is similar in function to the cell membrane of other animal cells. Myofibrils, one of the smaller functional units within a myocyte, consist of long, thin (approximately 1/1000 millimeter) chain proteins. The smallest functional unit of a muscle fiber, a sarcomere, contains the actin and myosin protein filaments responsible for the mechanical process of muscle contractions.

4. C: The sinoatrial (SA) node is the initiator of the rhythmic electrical impulses of the cardiac cycle. The SA node is located in the upper wall of the right atrium and contains a small locus of specialized muscle fibers that naturally generate action potentials.

5. C: On an EKG, the T-wave corresponds to the recovery of the ventricles from depolarization, which is also known as repolarization. On the reading, this occurs after the QRS complex – the graphical representation of ventricular depolarization and contraction.

6. C: Capillaries are responsible for the exchange of nutrients, hormones, oxygen, fluids, and electrolytes between the blood and interstitial fluid in tissues. Hemoglobin helps carry oxygen and iron in circulating red blood cells. Arterioles and venules are intermediately-sized blood vessels, but their walls are too thick for cellular-level exchange.

7. A: During the excitation-contraction coupling phase, an electrical discharge at the muscle starts a series of chemical events on the surface of muscle cells. This causes the release of calcium ions (CA^{2+}) from the sarcoplasmic reticulum, resulting in the increase in intracellular calcium, which helps the myosin globular heads attach to the thin actin filaments.

8. C: Heavy breathing requires the movement of the ribs to accommodate lung expansion. The muscles that help to elevate the ribs during inspiration are the external intercostals, sternocleidomastoids, anterior serrati, and scalenes. Rectus abdominis is a group of superficial abdominal muscles that do not affect rib movement.

9. B: The transverse plane is a horizontal plane that divides the body into upper and lower regions. A backhand or forehand tennis swing occurs in the horizontal plane at approximately the midsection of the body. Punting a football and throwing a shot put are movements that occur in the sagittal plane, and dribbling a soccer ball takes place mostly in the frontal plane.

10. D: The supinator is responsible for rotation of the forearm, helping to pivot the radius on the ulna; the other three muscles are responsible for the rotation of the arm.

11. C: A third-class lever has resistive force (F_r) at one end of the lever, muscle force (F_M)is applied in the middle of the lever, and the fulcrum is at the opposite end. During a bicep curl, the F_r is the barbell (in the hand), the F_M is the contraction of the biceps, and the elbow joint is the fulcrum in the middle. There are few physiologic examples of first- and second-class levers, although the head on the neck is a first-class lever, and the metatarsophalangeal joint serves as the fulcrum of a second-class lever when one stands on his or her toes.

12. C: Elbow extension and wrist flexion are movements that both take place in the sagittal plane, which cuts through the anterior and posterior of the body, dividing the body into right and left sides. Shoulder abduction and neck left tilt movements both occur in the frontal plane.

13. B: Ankle inversion is required for soccer dribbling to help expose the inside of the foot for an adequate kicking surface. Inversion takes place in the frontal plane, which runs through the center of the body from side to side, dividing the body into front and back halves.

14.A:

Name of Fascicular Arrangement	Structure of Fascicular Arrangement	Muscle Example
Circular	Fascicles are arranged in a concentric ring	Obicularis oris (muscles surrounding mouth)
Convergent (sometimes called radiate)	Muscle has a broad origin and is fan- or triangular-shaped	Pectoralis major; gluteus medius
Parallel/longitudinal	Long axis of fascicles are parallel to long axis of muscle	Rectus abdominis
Unipennate	Short fascicles insert obliquely into only one side of tendon	Extensor digitorum longus; tibialis posterior
Bipennate	Fascicles insert into opposite sides of one central tendon	Rectus femoris
Multipennate	Tendon branches within the muscle	Deltoid
Fusiform	Spindle-shaped muscles	Biceps brachii

15. D: Isometric contractions occur when a muscle generates a force but is unable to shorten because the resistance force is greater than the generated force. In this situation, force is still generated, but the action does not cause movement or external work. Shortening does occur with concentric contractions, while eccentric contractions are lengthening contractions, and isotonic contractions occur when there is no change in tension, but length may change.

16. B: Power (measured in watts [W]) is the rate that work is performed and, accordingly, is calculated as work divided by time. Power can also be calculated as the force applied to an object multiplied by velocity. Choice *A*, force × distance, is the equation for work.

17. D: The phosphagen system is the primary energy system stressed when using a work-to-rest ratio of 1:12 to 1:20. Additionally, an exercise duration of 5-10 seconds that uses 90-100 percent of maximum effort is used to stress this system. Energy is rapidly generated with this system because there are very few steps in the process, but only a small amount of energy is released, which is why exercise duration fueled with this pathway is so brief.

18. B: Fats have a greatest capacity for ATP production compared to carbohydrates and protein.

19. B: The electron transport chain (ETC) uses two pyruvate molecules, six molecules of nicotinamide adenine dinucleotide (NADH), two flavin adenine dinucleotide ($FADH_2$), and hydrogen atoms to produce ATP. Hydrogen atoms form a proton concentration gradient down the ETC and provide the energy required to produce ATP. NADH and $FADH_2$ molecules rephosphorylate ADP to ATP via the ETC, with each NADH producing three ATP molecules and each $FADH_2$ producing two ATP molecules.

20. C: Oxidative phosphorylation is the process of ATP being resynthesized via the actions of the ETC. The ETC is not part of the phosphagen system.

21. B: The primary source of ATP during low-intensity activity and while the body is at rest is the oxidative system. This system utilizes carbohydrates and fats as substrates. Glycolysis and the phosphagen system are both anaerobic systems that supply energy during high-intensity exercise.

22. C: One molecule of glucose results in the net production of thirty-eight ATP materials. Complete glycolysis with oxidation accounts for ten ATP molecules, and the Krebs cycle and ETC produce thirty ATP molecules for a total ATP production of forty molecules. Two molecules of ATP are invested in glycolysis, so the net production is thirty-eight ATP molecules.

23. D: Catabolism is the process of breaking large molecules into smaller molecules to release energy for work. Carbohydrates and fats are catabolized to provide energy for exercise and daily activities. Anabolism synthesizes larger molecules from smaller constituent building blocks. Bioenergetics and metabolism are more general terms involving overall energy production and usage.

24. C: When sufficient oxygen is available, pyruvate is transported to the mitochondrial matrix to take part in the Krebs cycle. Pyruvate is converted to acetyl-coenzyme A (acetyl-CoA) by pyruvate dehydrogenase, resulting in the loss of CO_2, and the acetyl-CoA enters the Krebs cycle to resynthesize ATP. Under anaerobic conditions, fermentation occurs, and pyruvate is converted to lactate, and NADH is reduced to NAD+.

25. A: Cortisol is a glucocorticoid secreted by the adrenal cortex. The other structures listed also secrete hormones, but not cortisol.

26. D: Epinephrine is a catecholamine secreted by the adrenal medulla and is involved in the fight-or-fight response to stress. Testosterone, growth hormone, and insulin-like growth factor are the primary anabolic hormones. Anabolic hormones help the body with anabolic functions like synthesizing larger compounds from smaller constituent parts.

27. C: Cardiac output is not impacted by testosterone. Testosterone increases protein synthesis, muscle and bone growth, the rate of cellular metabolism, and the production of red blood cells.

28. A: Growth hormone concentration levels can be increased acutely by performing three high-intensity sets of each resistance exercise with short rest periods between sets.

29. A: Epinephrine and norepinephrine are catecholamines that increase the blood flow to muscles due to vasodilation. They also elevate blood pressure, increase the rate of muscle contraction, increase energy availability, enhance metabolic enzymatic activity, and increase the rate of testosterone secretion.

30. C: Acute increases in serum testosterone concentrations can be achieved by using heavy resistance loads of 85-95 percent of 1RM. Additionally, performing exercises that involve large-muscle groups (such as squats, dead lift, and power clean), completing moderate- to high-exercise volumes by performing multiple exercises or multiple sets, and utilizing short rest intervals of 30-60 seconds can also result in higher serum testosterone concentrations.

31. B: Overtraining syndrome is associated with blunted increases in pituitary hormones including growth hormone, so an increased level of growth hormone is not a symptom of overtraining syndrome.

32. C: The anterior pituitary gland secretes growth hormone and has a significant influence on the metabolic system and energy availability. Growth hormone has numerous other physiological functions including decreasing glucose utilization and glycogen synthesis, enhancing the function of immune cells, increasing availability of glucose and amino acids, and increasing collagen synthesis and cartilage growth.

33. C: The characteristics of mechanical load that stimulate bone growth are the speed of loading, the intensity of the load, and the direction of the force. In accordance to Wolff's Law, bone adapts to the stresses (or lack thereof) placed upon it. Type of load is not identified as a specific component of mechanical load needed to stimulate bone growth.

34. B: As part of the neural response to high-intensity resistance training, the recruitment of motor units in an orderly manner is controlled by the size principle. The size principle is a method used by motor units to modulate force production, and it is dependent upon how many motor units are activated. If more force is needed for an activity, a greater number of motor units will be recruited. The smallest motor units are recruited first, and as more force is needed, larger motor units are sequentially activated. These strategies are designed to help the body be as efficient as possible.

35. B: Tendon stiffness increases in response to anaerobic training, and therefore, tendons become less flexible. While this may sound negative, stiffer tendons have a better mechanical advantage and are more efficient at transferring muscular work to the connected joints to produce powerful movements. High-intensity anaerobic training causes connective tissue growth and structural changes. Specific changes within a tendon include an increase in collagen fibril diameter, number, and packing density.

36. C: Choice C is the only answer containing the three correct functions while excluding option III (increased peripheral blood flow during the set). Muscular contractions greater than 20 percent of maximum voluntary contraction slow peripheral blood flow during a set, but during rest, blood flow increases to levels above baseline. Acute anaerobic exercise increases cardiac output, heart rate, stroke volume, and systolic blood pressure.

37. C: Ventilation significantly increases during each resistance exercise set; however, ventilation is greatest during the first minute of recovery from the set. This is termed excess post-oxygen consumption (EPOC) and serves to help the body return to homeostasis after the work is performed. By increasing ventilation rate, more oxygen enters the body to help perfuse tissues, resynthesize hormones and metabolic intermediates such as creatine phosphate, buffer lactate, etc.

38. A: Anaerobic training increases tendon stiffness, which is directly associated with greater muscular recoil and power production because a stiffer tendon is better able to transfer forces from muscular contractions to the joints the muscles control, resulting in better efficiency and, thus, higher power. Flexibility is not improved. Decreased ability to withstand tensile forces and risk of injury do not necessarily increase in accordance to tendon stiffness, but depend on many other factors such as biomechanics, proper load selection, fatigue, training status, and hydration.

39. D: To avoid developing low bone mineral density, athletes should participate in weight-bearing exercise, regular resistance exercise training sessions, and other dry-land exercises. The cyclist and swimmer both participate in non–weight-bearing sport activities. The swimmer runs during off-season and has a regular resistance training program; both activities can help to build and maintain bone mineral density. The distance cyclist has only one resistance training session per week. The cyclist is the athlete most likely to have the lowest level of bone mineral density.

40. C: Aerobic programs that stimulate bone growth must be high-intensity weight-bearing activities such as running and aerobics. Bone growth is not stimulated by non–weight-bearing activities, so although aerobic exercise such as swimming and cycling provide many health benefits, they do not promote bone growth.

41. A: Resting heart rate is an adaptation that athletes can easily assess by measuring their pulse upon waking in the morning. Aerobic training can improve the ability of the heart to pump blood at rest by increasing chamber size, cardiac muscle strength (particularly in the ventricles), and the afterload, which is the amount of blood returned to the chamber during diastole (relaxation or filling), resulting in a greater stroke volume of blood ejected per beat. These factors together account for the bradycardia of highly-trained endurance athletes.

42. A: VO$_2$ max or maximal oxygen consumption can be reduced by 4-14 percent over 4 weeks of reduced training stimulus or rest and 6-20 percent over a down period of more than 4 weeks.

43. A: Increased blood lactate concentrations is not an adaptation to aerobic endurance training. There are numerous cardiovascular responses that occur in response to an acute bout of aerobic exercise. These physiological changes include increases in the following: stroke volume and heart rate and resultant cardiac output, systolic blood pressure, oxygen uptake into tissues, blood flow to working muscles, and vasodilation of blood vessels.

44. C: The athlete can control various health behaviors that can impact adaptations to aerobic endurance training. While genetic potential can significantly impact training adaptions, maximal aerobic power decreases with age, and men typically have greater aerobic power than women, athletes cannot control these factors.

45. C: Decreased muscle glycogen, not increased muscle glycogen, has been identified as a sign of aerobic overtraining syndrome.

46. B: Training age refers to the length of time that the youth athlete has participated in a formal, supervised resistance training program. Both biological and chronological age should be considered in the development of the program; however, these factors do not provide information about potential adaptations to resistance training achieved from past training programs.

47. C: While strength and conditioning professionals should never treat youth athletes as miniature adults, they should provide easily understandable, quality instruction and progress athletes at a conservative but appropriate rate. Youth athletes are typically new to the sport and formal training programs, so they should receive thorough verbal and then visual demonstrations of appropriate resistance exercise techniques, utilizing kinesthetic learning and parts practice as well. The program should start with low resistance and use sets of six to fifteen repetitions for a variety of single- and multi-joint exercises. This training should involve two to three training sessions occurring on nonconsecutive days each week and focus on proper form and technique, fun, and positive feedback.

48. B: Changes in muscle hypertrophy may be partially responsible for increased strength, but strength gains are primarily due to neurological factors resulting from nervous system development. Factors include increased motor unit recruitment, activation, synchronization, and firing.

49. C: When considering absolute strength, females have about two-thirds that of males, with lower body strength being closer to that of males as compared to upper body strength. When strength is considered relative to body weight, lower body strength is similar in the sexes; however, the relative upper body strength of females is still less than males. Importantly, when strength is expressed relative to the cross-sectional area of a muscle, no strength differences exist between males and females, indicating that muscle quality is not sex specific.

50. A: Although females are six times more likely than males to experience an ACL tear, this injury is not part of the female athlete triad. The triad stems from disordered eating, which leads to insufficient caloric intake for expenditure. This causes a cessation in menstruation (amenorrhea), and overtime, this reduces bone mineral density due to the lack of estrogen needed for adequate calcification of bones.

51. B: A bone mineral density level between 1 and 2.5 standard deviations below the young adult comparator group (a negative standard deviation) indicates that the woman has osteopenia. Osteoporosis is defined as a bone mineral density with a standard deviation of -2.5 standard or more, indicating it is well below the normal range for young adults. Sarcopenia refers to the loss of muscle mass, causing decreases in strength and power.

52. D: Any training program developed for an older adult should be multidimensional with aerobic and resistance exercise and balance training to maximize improvement of neuromuscular function. Developing a resistance training program for older adults is similar to developing a program for younger adults. Additionally, the strength and conditioning professional should take a detailed medical history, ask about previous aerobic and resistance training programs, and have the older adult complete a risk assessment questionnaire. In most circumstances, it may be appropriate for the older adult to have a medical examination from his or her primary physician and get a signed form stating the older adult can participate in the program.

53. D: Robert's behavior is driven by intrinsic motivation. He loves the game, gets personal satisfaction out of participating, and is continually working on new skills and improving. With achievement motivation, athletes are looking to master a specific task, outperform competitors or otherwise achieve excellence, and overcome obstacles. Extrinsic motivation typically comes in the form of individualized rewards such as praise from coaches and teammates, medals, social acceptance, avoidance of punishment, the drive for positive reinforcement, and other sources outside of the athlete. The construct of outcome motivation does not exist.

54. B: The ideal performance state is referred to as "the zone" in many sporting applications. It is characterized by a sense of personal strength and effortless performance and control, increased attentiveness and focus on the activity at hand, confidence and feelings of capability, and mental clarity. Arousal that is too high leads to anxiety and can impair performance.

55. D: Somatic anxiety is the negative physical perceptions of anxiety such as increased heart rate, nervous stomach, and sweaty palms. Anxiety is perceived as a negative emotional state characterized by worry, nervousness, apprehension, and fear. The thought process responsible for the perception of arousal as negative is a result of cognitive anxiety, while its counterpart – somatic anxiety – is the perception of physical symptoms.

56. C: Progressive muscular relaxation is used by athletes to control anxiety. It is particularly useful for controlling pre-competition levels of somatic and cognitive anxiety and regulating levels of physical and psychological arousal. This relaxation technique consists of tightening and relaxing muscle groups throughout the body in succession until the entire body is relaxed.

57. B: Selective attention is the ability to focus on relevant, task-oriented cues while ignoring other stimuli and thoughts unrelated to the athletic performance. The basketball player blocking out external distractions while focusing on the free-throw shot is utilizing selective attention.

58. B: Self-efficacy (SE) is the athlete's perception of his or her ability to perform a situation-specific task successfully. There are numerous sources that influence SE, especially an athlete's past performance accomplishments and experiences. The swimmer's successful performance in preseason is an example of past performance accomplishments. Vicarious experience refers to the athlete watching someone similar achieve a successful performance and then decide that he or she, too, can have a successful performance. Verbal persuasion refers to encouragement from coaches, athletes, teammates, oneself, and other external sources. Physiological states refer to whether an athlete interprets his or her arousal as facilitative or detrimental.

59. A: This question requires understanding the characteristics of long jump and applying the concepts for motor skill practice. Given that long jump has a low degree of interdependence of parts but is highly complex, it is best to use parts practice. Sarah's coach can break down the event into several sections (e.g., the run, the take-off, body position after take-off). The whole practice method teaches the skill in its entirety and is better reserved for skills that are not very complex but are highly organized, or that have a high degree of interdependence, in that they can't be easily broken into steps because all parts or movements go together. Discovery and divided discovery are two types of instructions. Guided discovery gives less information to the athlete than explicit instruction but provides a generalized description of the overall movement. Discovery provides no instructions. Instead, it simply gives the overall goal of a movement.

60. D: John's goal is a process goal because it focuses on a specific action (maintenance of running technique in final 400 meters of race), is under his control, and successful achievement of the goal is dependent upon the amount of effort he puts in to successfully achieve the goal. An athlete has little control over an outcome goal, which typically is an event outcome, because he or she is unable to control the efforts and abilities of the competitors.

Nutrition

Nutritional Factors Affecting Health and Performance

Meal planning applications
There are a number of health- and performance-related applications that can be used for meal planning. Some health- and performance-related applications that can be used for nutrition include the United States Department of Agriculture (USDA) Food Patterns, the DASH (Dietary Approaches to Stop Hypertension) Eating Plan, MyPlate, food exchanges, and the glycemic index.

USDA Food Patterns
There are three USDA Food Patterns included in the 2015-2020 Dietary Guidelines: Healthy U.S. Style Eating, Healthy Mediterranean Style Eating, and Healthy Vegetarian Style Eating. One eating pattern is not necessarily superior to another, but rather more of a preference; however, a vegetarian lifestyle has been associated with a decreased risk for some chronic diseases such as heart disease and certain cancers. The USDA Food Patterns are all based on systematic review from scientific research, food pattern modeling, and analysis of intake of the U.S. population. Each USDA Food Pattern is based on the five food groups—vegetables, fruits, grains, dairy, and protein—and can be customized to meet an individual's needs based on age, sex, height, weight, and level of physical activity.

The Healthy U.S. Style Eating Pattern is based on typical foods consumed in Americans' diets with a focus on nutrient-dense foods in portions that are appropriate for the desired caloric intake. The Healthy Mediterranean Style Eating Pattern is based on the Healthy U.S. Style Eating Pattern but adjusted to align with the eating patterns of the Mediterranean diet, which have been associated with positive health outcomes. Specifically, the Healthy Mediterranean Style Eating Pattern has more fruit and seafood but less dairy than the U.S. Style Eating Pattern. The Healthy Vegetarian Style Eating Pattern is also based on the Healthy U.S. Style Eating Pattern but is adjusted to reflect the eating habits of self-reported vegetarians, as identified in the National Health and Nutrition Examination Survey (NHANES).

DASH Eating Plan
The DASH Eating Plan is based on clinical research trials, which found that the plan helped individuals lower their blood pressure and low-density lipoprotein (LDL) cholesterol and improve heart health, while meeting nutrient requirements. The DASH Eating Plan emphasizes whole grains, poultry, fish, and nuts along with food sources of potassium, calcium, and magnesium. Individuals are encouraged to consume as much as seven to eight servings of grains and four to five servings of fruits and vegetables per day on a 2000-calorie diet. Individuals using the DASH Eating Plan may need to gradually increase the intake of whole grains, fruits, and vegetables, since the increased fiber of these foods can lead to bloating and diarrhea.

MyPlate
MyPlate is a tool developed by the USDA based on the five food groups and healthy eating, focused on variety, appropriate portion sizes, nutrient-dense foods, and low saturated fat, sodium, and added sugar intake. The MyPlate Daily Checklist and the SuperTracker are two specific online tools that allow individuals to customize nutrition planning for their specific needs.

Food Exchanges
Food exchanges are used for meal planning purposes, especially for those with diabetes and/or seeking weight loss. Food exchanges divide food into six categories based on the amount of carbohydrate, fat, and protein they contain: starches/breads, fruits, milk, vegetables, meat, and fat.

- Starches and breads contain 15 grams of carbohydrate and 3 grams of protein per exchange with 80 calories.

- Fruits contain 15 grams of carbohydrate per exchange with 60 calories.

- Milk exchanges contain 12 grams of carbohydrate; 8 grams of protein; 3-8 grams of fat depending on whether the milk exchange is a low-, medium-, or high-fat choice; and 90-150 calories depending on the fat content.

- Vegetable exchanges contain 5 grams of carbohydrate per serving with 25 calories.

- Meat exchanges contain 7 grams of protein per ounce and 0-8 grams of fat, depending on whether the source of the meat exchange is very lean, lean, medium fat, or high fat with a range of 35-100 calories.

- Fat exchanges provide 5 grams of fat and 45 calories.

Glycemic Index
Finally, the glycemic index and glycemic load offer insight as to how foods affect blood glucose and insulin levels. Glycemic index and load can be useful tools in meal planning to help individuals better understand the impact specific foods may have on their blood sugar. Carbohydrate counting may also be a useful tool in helping individuals monitor and understand the impact various carbohydrates have on their blood sugar.

Meal Planning Approaches
Each of these meal planning approaches are useful in working with athletes to guide them toward healthy eating. The most appropriate meal planning approach depends on the athlete's nutrition goals and personal preferences. For example, an athlete wanting to lower blood pressure and blood lipids may be best served with the DASH approach. Another athlete who would like to adopt a vegetarian lifestyle may be more interested in using the USDA Healthy Vegetarian Style Eating Pattern, while an athlete interested in lowering blood sugar might be interested in food exchanges and/or the glycemic index as a meal planning approach.

Nutritional Needs of Athletes
Nutritional requirements for athletes are typically higher than nonathletes and vary depending on the type of activity.

Carbohydrates
Carbohydrates provide 4 kilocalories per gram and are a major source of fuel for the body during moderate- and high-intensity exercise, up to 2 hours in duration. Beyond approximately this duration, stores deplete and the body relies on fatty acid metabolism for sustained energy. Carbohydrates are used for energy immediately, if needed, but excess carbohydrates are converted to glycogen and stored in skeletal muscles and the liver or converted to fat if the body's glycogen stores are full. The amount of glycogen the body can store is influenced by a variety of factors including physical training status, basal metabolic rate, body size, and eating habits, but in general, the body can store about 15 grams per

kilogram of body weight. In general, athletes should consume about 6-10 grams of carbohydrate per kilogram of body weight daily, depending on the intensity, duration, and frequency of their training as well as their current health and physical goals.

Protein
Like carbohydrates, protein provides 4 kilocalories per gram. Protein, which consists of amino acids, is used to support the body in the development of tissues, enzymes, and hormones and to rebuild and repair muscles after exercise. In general, protein recommendations for athletes fall in the range of 1.5-2.0 grams per kilogram of body weight daily, depending on the type, duration, and frequency of exercise. Excessive consumption of protein does not lead to increased muscle mass because protein in excess of physiologic needs is converted and stored as fat.

Fat
Fat provides 9 kilocalories per gram and contributes significantly to resting energy requirements as well as requirements during low-intensity and long-duration exercise. Fats can be divided into two basic categories: saturated and unsaturated. Saturated fats, which are primarily found in animal sources, include butyric, lauric, myristic, palmitic, and stearic acid, while unsaturated fats typically come from plant sources such as soybeans, nuts, seeds, olives, and avocados. Fats should comprise at least 15% of the total caloric intake; as much as 30%-40% can be acceptable, depending on the health, age, and needs of the individual. For athletes, an intake of 30% fat (10% saturated, 10% polyunsaturated, and 10% monounsaturated) aligns with dietary guidelines and should ensure an adequate – but not excessive – dietary intake.

The body's use of fat as an energy source during exercise depends on the length and intensity of the event and the athlete's fitness level. Generally speaking, two phenomena can describe an athlete's use of fat as an energy substrate during exercise: the crossover concept and the duration effect. The crossover concept refers to the fact that at lower intensities, the body is primarily using fat as a source of fuel, and as the intensity increases, the contribution of adenosine triphosphate (ATP) from carbohydrate metabolism increases. The duration effect is based on the principle that as the duration of the exercise bout increases, the body relies more heavily on fat, as carbohydrate stores deplete. Exactly how much of each fuel source is used also depends on the athlete's aerobic fitness; fitter athletes typically can store more glycogen but also use fat at higher intensities of exercise. Lastly, there is some evidence to suggest that women derive a greater percentage of their energy needs from fat, compared to men, at a given exercise workload.

Vitamins and Minerals
Vitamin and mineral needs of athletes may be increased, but typically can be met if a balanced, varied diet is consumed with foods such as lean meats/protein, fruits, vegetables, whole grains, and dairy. B vitamins such as thiamin, riboflavin, and niacin are required to support metabolic processes; vitamin D is required for calcium absorption, and vitamins C and E are required to mitigate stress oxidation in the body. Fat-soluble vitamins (A, D, E, and K) are stored in the body, so they should not be consumed in excessive quantities. If an athlete is not meeting their vitamins and minerals requirements through diet, a multivitamin-mineral supplement is needed. Such supplements will not directly improve athletic performance but will help to correct a nutrition deficiency if one is present, which may prevent illness or improve performance.

Sweating can lower electrolytes and minerals such as sodium, potassium, chloride, iron, calcium, phosphorus, and magnesium. Sodium and potassium help to regulate the body's water balance and also play a significant role in muscle contraction. Chloride also helps with fluid balance and nerve conductions. Iron plays an important role in the body's ability to transport and use oxygen, and calcium is critical for bone formation, nerve conduction, and muscle contraction. Phosphorus is involved in intramuscular oxidation processes, and magnesium helps support energy metabolism. Electrolytes (sodium, potassium, and chloride) and water need to be replaced during extended exercise, particularly in hot and humid environments, because they are lost in sweat.

Health Risk Factors Associated with Dietary Choices
Dietary choices affect health risks associated with some chronic health conditions.

Saturated fats
Saturated fat is associated with an increased risk for cardiovascular disease, so the Dietary Guidelines for Americans recommends consuming no more than 10% of caloric intake from saturated fats. An emphasis should be made on replacing saturated fats with unsaturated fats, especially polyunsaturated, as this substitution is associated with improved total and LDL cholesterol.

Triglycerides
Circulating triglycerides are also affected by diet. Limiting refined, sugary foods; replacing saturated fats with unsaturated fats; and increasing fiber intake can help to keep triglycerides in the normal range of less than 150 milligrams per deciliter. High triglycerides can lead to increased risk of heart disease and diabetes.

Trans fats
Trans fats are produced through a process called *hydrogenation,* which makes packaged foods (such as coffee creamer, snack foods, store-bought baked goods, vegetable shortening, stick margarines, fast foods, and refrigerated dough products) more shelf stable. In recent years, manufacturers have begun limiting or removing trans fats per the Food and Drug Administration regulatory requirements because these fats have been shown to pose a significant risk for heart disease and should be eliminated from the diet.

Cholesterol
Cholesterol is required for various physiological and structural functions, such as the production of cells and hormones. However, these requirements are met by the cholesterol produced in the body; little to no additional dietary cholesterol is needed. The upper limit for healthy levels of cholesterol is 200 milligrams per deciliter; high cholesterol is a risk factor for heart disease. Because recent research has failed to find a significant correlation between dietary intake and circulating cholesterol, the 2015-2020 Dietary Guidelines no longer contain recommendations that limit cholesterol intake to 300 milligrams per day. The Institute of Medicine (IOM) still recommends limiting the intake of cholesterol-laden foods such as high-fat meats and dairy, which also contain high amounts of saturated fat.

Calcium
Calcium plays important physiologic roles including vascular contraction, vasodilation, muscle contraction, and nerve impulse transmission. The majority of calcium in the body is stored in bones and teeth. To support bone mineral deposition and avoid bone resorption, it is important to have adequate calcium intake. This is especially true at certain stages of the life cycle, when bones are forming or have the tendency to demineralize, as well as for athletes, who may lose additional calcium through perspiration. Postmenopausal women, especially, need to obtain adequate amounts of calcium in the diet to decrease the risk for osteoporosis. Signs and symptoms of calcium deficiency may be absent or may include muscle weakness, cramping, and increased susceptibility to fractures. Recommended intake varies by gender and throughout the lifespan, with increases for females, adolescents, lactating mothers, and postmenopausal women.

Iron
Iron in the body is primarily combined with hemoglobin, in an iron-protein compound that increases the blood's oxygen-carrying capacity 65 times, as well as in muscle myoglobin. Intensive workout programs put individuals at risk for developing iron-deficiency anemia, which decreases aerobic capacity, since less oxygen can circulate to working tissues, leading to fatigue and reduced athletic performance. Other symptoms of iron-deficiency anemia include brittle nails, sluggishness, headaches, pale skin, and dizziness. Iron recommendations are 1.3-1.7 times higher for athletes than nonathletes and another 1.8 times higher for vegetarian athletes in comparison to those who consume animal protein, due to the lower bioavailability of nonheme iron sources in the vegetarian diet. The Recommended Dietary Allowance (RDA) for iron for men over the age of 18 is 8 milligrams per day; for women ages 19-50, 18 milligrams; for women ages 51 and older, it is also 8 milligrams per day. Females of childbearing age are at a higher risk for iron-deficiency anemia due to red blood cell loss during menstruation. Females often tend to consume less dietary iron as well. Endurance athletes may require additional iron due to foot-strike hemolysis, loss of hemoglobin in urine from strenuous training, and the small amount of iron lost in sweat. Heme sources of iron are more easily absorbed and include beef, pork, and beef liver. Nonheme sources include oatmeal, lentils, dark green leafy vegetables, and fortified cereals. Vitamin C intake can increase the absorption of iron in the small intestine; a glass of orange juice increases nonheme iron bioavailability by three times. It should be noted that excessive iron intake, especially in males, can be toxic.

Hydration and Electrolytes
The adult male body is about 60% water, while the female body is about 50%-55% water. As a result, less than optimal hydration status can affect health and performance. Dehydration can cause headaches, sluggishness, mood changes and loss of cognitive functioning, and muscle cramping. Decreased physical performance can occur with just a 2% loss in body weight from dehydration, and the risk of heat illness increases significantly with a fluid loss equaling 3% or more of body weight. During exercise, perspiration helps mitigate the increase in body temperature. During strenuous activity,

individuals can lose as much as 6%-10% of their body weight via sweating, depending on the type and duration of the activity. It is important to maintain adequate hydration before, during, and after exercise; the recommendation is 8-12 cups of water per day plus replacement of fluid loss during exercise. Individual needs may vary, but during exercise, about 6-8 ounces of fluid are usually needed every 15-20 minutes of activity. Within the context of adequate hydration, electrolyte balance must also be preserved. The five major electrolytes that are important to health are sodium, potassium, chloride, calcium, and magnesium. Sodium, which is needed to help maintain fluid balance, nerve function, muscle contractions, and acid-base balance, is the primary electrolyte lost in sweat and must be replaced. It is important to include sodium in fluids or food as part of the rehydration process after exercise so that overhydration, or hyponatremia, does not occur as a result of drinking water alone. Adding sodium to fluids also helps to improve the absorption of water and carbohydrates. Most commercial sports drinks are formulated to provide the optimal levels of sodium and carbohydrates in solution.

Children and seniors are particularly susceptible to dehydration during exercise. Children may be unware of the need to replace fluids during activity and may need longer to acclimate to increased temperatures. When children are exercising in hot environments, they should be well hydrated before activity and drink plenty of fluid afterward. Aging leads to decreased lean body mass and, over time, decreased body water. Seniors may also be at risk for dehydration because of decreased sensitivity to thirst and diminished ability of the kidneys to concentrate urine in the absence of adequate hydration.

Nutrient-dense versus caloric-dense foods

Nutrient-dense foods are rich in essential nutrients, vitamins, and minerals but low in calories, especially in comparison to calorically-dense or energy-dense foods. Calorically-dense foods provide few essential nutrients relative to the number of calories they provide. When focusing on weight loss or optimal health, it is important to focus on nutrient-dense foods. Sources of nutrient-dense foods include fresh vegetables and fruits, specifically dark green leafy vegetables like kale, spinach, and collard greens and fruits like berries, melon, mangoes, and citrus. Other nutrient-dense foods include lean sources of protein, dairy, legumes, and whole grains that have been enriched with vitamins and minerals. Calorically-dense foods include cookies, cakes, pastries, soda, chips, high-fat meats, and fast foods and other highly processed, highly caloric foods.

There are a number of systems that can be used in nutritional profiling or rating to support choosing nutrient-dense foods. Nutritional rating systems, which offer guidance on the nutritional value of food to make selection easier, differ from nutrition labeling, which provides detailed nutrient content on the specific food item according to serving size. Some nutritional rating systems include the Glycemic Index, the Guiding Star, Nutripoints, Nutrition IQ, the Naturally Nutrient Rich Score, the NuVal Nutritional Scoring System, the Aggregate Nutrient Density Index (ANDI), the ReViVer score, and the Points Food System by Weight Watchers. The Dietary Guidelines, to some extent, can also be considered a nutritional rating system.

Manipulating Food Choices and Training Methods to Maximize Performance

<u>Nutrition and Training Programs</u>
Nutrition and training strategies can be used to guide changes in body composition. However, a calorie deficit is needed to lose body fat, which is usually best accomplished through diet and exercise. Nutrition strategies for losing body fat include altering the macronutrient composition of the diet, increasing protein and fiber intake, reducing consumption of processed and fast food, consuming five to six small meals per day, creating a reasonable calorie deficit, and drinking plenty of water.

Altering Macronutrient Composition
Studies lasting about 6 months in duration have found that moderately decreasing carbohydrates, increasing protein, and getting enough healthy fat is more successful in decreasing body fat than simply limiting caloric intake. However, results are more equivocal during 12-month and longer-term studies. It is important to remember that total caloric intake does play a role in energy balance. One pound of body fat contains about 3500 kilocalories, so caloric intake and expenditure should be modified accordingly for weight loss goals. Macronutrient composition needs to be tailored to the individual based on body composition, health status, training, and goals, but a caloric distribution of about 40%-45% carbohydrate, 30%-35% protein, and 25% fat should reduce body fat when part of a diet with appropriate caloric intake.

Increasing Protein and Fiber Intake
Increasing protein helps to support muscle tissue and is necessary to increase lean body mass and metabolism. While the minimum RDA for individuals is 0.8 grams per kilogram of body weight, this is typically not enough for individuals who are seeking to maintain lean body mass while losing body fat. Protein requirements vary based on the type, duration, intensity of training, as well as fitness and health goals; however, most athletes need at least 1.0-1.7 grams per kilogram of body weight. Depending on the individual's eating preferences, the focus should be on lean sources of nutrient-dense protein such as beef, chicken, turkey, eggs, yogurt, fish, beans, and legumes. Since increasing fiber in the diet helps to increase satiety and fullness, plenty of fruits, vegetables, legumes, and whole grains should also be included.

Consuming Small Meals

Consuming five to six small meals per day helps prevent the metabolism from slowing, which is one of the primary reasons that excessively low-calorie diets should be avoided. To help with satiety and blood glucose control, protein should be consumed at each of the small meals. While modified fasting diets have been shown to be effective in weight loss, fasting diets should not be used long-term because of their effect on slowing the metabolism.

Drinking Water

Drinking plenty of water helps to ensure adequate hydration and plasma levels for circulating nutrients and eliminating waste more effectively. As mentioned, the body is composed of about 60% water, so hydration is essential for optimal health and athletic performance. The Institute of Medicine recommends about 13 cups of fluid per day for men and about 9 cups per day for women. All fluids in the diet can be counted toward daily fluid requirements. Individual requirements vary depending on health, activity, and environment, but athletes should be mindful to replace fluids lost from sweating. To ensure fluid replacement after exercise is adequate, athletes should determine their sweat rate and fluid loss by weighing themselves before and after exercise.

Increasing Lean Body Mass Through Training

Strategies for increasing lean body mass through exercise include weight training and cardio interval training. Individuals require a specific program depending on their goals, but to increase lean body mass, progressive resistance training should be a part of the regimen at least three times per week. High-intensity interval training (HIIT), which involves alternating bouts of high-intensity activity with rest, is also effective for building lean body mass. Because it increases post-exercise oxygen consumption, HIIT can increase caloric expenditure and reduce body fat.

Composition and Timing of Nutrient and Fluid Intake

The body's preferred source of energy comes from muscles and liver glycogen stores; however, these stores are limited and not sufficient for sustained high-intensity athletic performance. Nutrient timing refers to effectively altering the content and timing of dietary intake – particularly carbohydrates and protein – to deliver optimal health and performance. Nutrient timing can involve the use of whole foods, isolated nutrients from food sources, as well as synthetic compounds, and may vary by sport and among individuals. Research results have found that appropriate nutrient timing provides superior health and athletic performance compared to unplanned or traditional intake strategies.

Carbohydrate Loading

Carbohydrate loading is one specific nutrient timing strategy used by endurance athletes to help maximize glycogen stores. Recall that glycogen is stored carbohydrates in the muscles and liver and is the body's preferred fuel source during moderate- and high-intensity activity. For optimal performance, it is important for athletes to have adequate stores of glycogen before beginning an endurance activity lasting 2 hours or more. To accomplish carbohydrate loading, athletes first deplete their carbohydrate stores through reducing carbohydrate intake while maintaining exercise volume and intensity about 5 days out from the event and then increase carbohydrate intake (to 8-10 grams per kilogram of body weight) and taper training volume for several days just before the event. Carbohydrate loading is typically recommended for activities that last longer than 120 minutes because this is roughly the threshold for depleting glycogen stores during intense exercise.

Nutrient Timing—Before, During, And After

Nutrient timing recommendations can be divided into three categories: before, during, and after exercise recommendations. The International Society of Sports Nutrition (ISSN) recommends 8-10 grams of carbohydrate per kilogram of body weight alone or with protein before resistance exercise to maximize glycogen stores. During exercise, 30-60 grams of carbohydrate per hour in 8-16 ounces of fluid should be consumed every 15 minutes or so. The addition of protein at a ratio of 3-4 grams of carbohydrate per 1 gram of protein may support endurance and the formation of glycogen after the activity. For resistance exercise, the intake of carbohydrate alone or combined with protein improves muscle glycogen, minimizes muscle damage, and supports strength training efforts. Within 30 minutes after exercise, ingestion of carbohydrate and protein helps to rebuild glycogen stores; the ISSN recommends an intake of 8-10 grams per kilogram of body weight for carbohydrate and 0.2-0.5 grams per kilogram of body weight of protein in the post-exercise meal. The ISSN posits that the intake of essential amino acids (EAAs) stimulates muscle protein synthesis; adding carbohydrates to the amino acid intake may further help increase muscle protein synthesis. Finally, during bouts of continuous, prolonged strength training, consuming carbohydrate and protein together has been demonstrated to improve strength and body composition, again, typically in a 3 to 1 or 4 to 1 ratio of carbohydrates to protein.

The Effects of Nutrition on Exercise

The primary nutritional factors that affect muscular endurance, hypertrophy, strength, and aerobic are carbohydrates and protein.

Carbohydrates

Carbohydrates provide fuel for neurons and red blood cells. Carbohydrates are also important for muscle contraction and because a state of positive energy balance is required to prevent muscle catabolism for energy. Athletes usually need about 55%-65% of their total calorie intake to come from carbohydrates to support activity and meet metabolic and physiologic demands.

Protein

Once the diet contains adequate carbohydrate to promote positive energy balance, adequate protein needs to be addressed to maintain a positive nitrogen balance. Nitrogen balance is usually addressed via laboratory analysis and entails comparing nitrogen intake and output. Individual intake requirements vary based on the type, intensity, and duration of activity and training, but athletes typically need a protein intake of about 1.5-2.0 grams per kilogram of body weight to maintain a positive nitrogen balance. Endurance athletes need additional protein to help support energy needs and to facilitate the repair and recovery after activity. Athletes focused on increasing strength and hypertrophy need more protein during the early stages of a training program; as muscles adapt to training, needs may decrease.

Protein is essential in the diet and is needed to support the building of connective tissue, cell membranes, and the development of muscle. Protein consists of amino acids, and there are 20 amino acids used in the body. Essential amino acids (EAAs) are required through the diet, since they cannot be synthesized in the body, and the nine of them include isoleucine, leucine, lysine, methionine, phenylalanine, threonine, tryptophan, valine, and histidine. This last one, histidine, was originally thought to only be essential for infants, but more recent studies have found that it is indeed essential for adults as well. Therefore, the discrepancy between sources that report that there are only eight EAAs and current ones typically is caused by more outdated resources failing to recognize the newer research that the adult body also does not produce histidine in sufficient quantities (so it must be consumed). There are also seven conditional amino acids that cannot be sufficiently produced in the body, so they should come from the diet: arginine, cysteine, glutamine, proline, taurine, glycine, and tyrosine. There are five non-EAAs: alanine, asparagine, aspartic acid, glutamic acid, and serine. These amino acids can be produced by the body so are not required in the diet.

Protein can be categorized as complete or incomplete. Complete proteins contain all of the EAAs, while incomplete proteins do not. Protein that comes from animal sources is usually complete and contains all of the EAAs, while incomplete proteins typically come from plant sources and do not contain all the EAAs. Proteins that have a higher amount of the EAAs are considered to have a higher amino acid profile. Good sources of animal protein include meat (beef, chicken, turkey, pork, and lamb), eggs, fish/seafood (tuna, crab, shrimp, lobster), and dairy (milk, yogurt, and cheese). Sources of plant-based protein include grains (brown rice, spelt, quinoa, amaranth, oatmeal), legumes (beans, peas, and lentils—pinto, black kidney, garbanzo, edamame, and tofu), and nuts and seeds (peanut butter, almond butter, peanuts, almonds, pistachios, walnuts, pecans, pumpkin seeds, and sunflower seeds).

Signs, Symptoms, and Behaviors Associated With Eating Disorders and Altered Eating Habits

Signs and Symptoms of Eating Disorders
Disordered eating is an umbrella term used to describe abnormal eating patterns and behaviors. Disordered eating behaviors include binge eating, dieting that can be described as abnormal or obsessive, regularly skipping meals, self-induced vomiting, calorie counting to a level that is obsessive, having a self-worth tied to physique, misusing diuretics and laxatives, and unhealthy fasting or restrictive eating. The root cause of an eating disorder may vary from one individual to another, but it is believed that eating disorders can be attributed to genetics, environment, social, and cultural factors. An eating disorder is a mental illness with a set of specific diagnostic criteria as described in the *Diagnostic and Statistical Manual of Mental Disorders* (DSM) published by the American Psychiatric Association, a professional association of psychiatric physicians. The most recent version of the DSM is the DSM-5, published in 2013, and it specifies four types of eating disorders: anorexia nervosa (AN), bulimia nervosa (BN), binge eating disorder (BED), and other eating disorders.

Anorexia Nervosa
Anorexia nervosa (AN) is characterized by consistently restricting caloric intake to keep body weight at least 15% lower than would be healthy for age, sex, development, and health; an intense fear of becoming overweight or obese; and having a distorted self-image of body weight or shape. Historically, AN has been more prevalent in females, although more recent studies indicate that adolescent females and males suffer from the disease equally. AN can further be classified into two subtypes: restricting and binge eating. Individuals who exhibit behavior of restricting AN limit certain food groups and/or their amounts, obsessively count calories, skip meals, and are obsessive in their attempt to adhere to guidance and rules governing consumption. Individuals with AN who exhibit binge eating behavior may also restrict certain food groups and quantities, but also display binging and purging behaviors. Binge eating involves eating a large amount of food and feeling a sense of loss of control while doing so; purging involves self-induced tactics to rid the body of food such as vomiting; using laxatives, diuretics, and enemas; or participating in excessive exercise.

Bulimia Nervosa
In bulimia nervosa (BN), similar to AN, individuals typically have a distorted self-image of body shape, weight, or size. Other behaviors characterized by BN include binge eating large amounts of food while feeling a sense of lack of control, self-induced vomiting, and misusing laxatives, diuretics, or enemas to prevent weight gain. In individuals with BN, the binge eating behavior occurs at least weekly for 3 months. Bulimia nervosa can further be categorized into purging and non-purging type behavior. Purging behaviors involve tactics to remove food from the body, while non-purging behaviors involve restricting food or engaging in excessive exercise to compensate for food that has been ingested.

Binge Eating Disorder

Binge eating disorder (BED) is characterized by persistent binge eating, feeling a sense of distress when binging, or binging on average weekly for 3 months. Binge eating is closely related to BN, but individuals do not engage in purging or other compensatory behaviors that would eliminate food from their bodies.

Other Eating Disorders

Other eating disorders are now classified in the DSM-5 as other specified feeding or eating disorder (OSFED) or unspecified feeding or eating disorder (UFED). These two categories are intended to recognize disordered eating behaviors that do not clearly align with other diagnosed and defined eating disorders. Night eating syndrome, which entails recurrent episodes of eating at night, is one example of an OSFED.

Effects of Eating Disorders on the Body and Performance

Physiological changes can occur as a result of disordered eating, putting individuals at risk for other health issues. Physical signs and symptoms that may be associated with AN and its behaviors include rapid weight loss, mineral and electrolyte imbalances, amenorrhea in females, decreased sex drive, fainting or dizziness, hypothermia, consistently feeling cold even in warm weather, bloating, constipation, food intolerances, fatigue, low energy level, changes in the face including sunken eyes, and the development of fine hair on the face and body. Health concerns associated with AN and its behaviors include anemia, immune compromise, gastrointestinal issues, amenorrhea in females, increased risk of infertility in men and women, renal failure, osteoporosis, cardiovascular issues, and ultimately, death.

Signs and symptoms that may be associated with BN include frequent change in weight; physical signs associated with vomiting including facial swelling, knuckle calluses, tooth decay, and bad breath; chronic sore throat; bloating, constipation, and food intolerances; amenorrhea; fainting or dizziness; and tiredness. Health concerns associated with BN include dehydration; gastrointestinal reflux, heartburn, and ulcers; slowed or irregular heart beat; electrolyte imbalances; and heart failure.

BED can lead to weight gain and obesity, high blood pressure, high cholesterol, kidney failure, osteoarthritis, diabetes, stroke, gallbladder disease, irregular menstrual cycle, skin disorders, heart disease, and some cancers.

As a result of disordered eating, individuals can develop physiological issues that lead to health problems. These health problems can lead to a variety of conditions that can compromise athletic performance and even lead to death. Youth and collegiate athletes who develop disordered eating are at even greater risk of injury and physiological complications, since growth and development may be affected by disordered eating. Female athletes are also at risk for the Female Athlete Triad—a combination of energy deficiency and/or disordered eating, irregular menstrual cycles or amenorrhea, and osteoporosis or bone mineral loss.

Treatment for Eating Disorders

Disordered eating is a complex mental illness that requires early detection and treatment by qualified health care professionals. As such, coaches and trainers need to be cognizant of the signs and symptoms of disordered eating and refer individuals in need of intervention to appropriate and qualified health care professionals. The complexity of the illnesses requires a multidisciplinary approach with a team of health care professionals such as a physician, psychologist, psychiatrist, social worker, and registered dietitian who have experience and expertise in working with individuals with disordered eating.

When individuals need to change their behavior, as in disordered eating, it's important to understand that change is a process and that individuals often move through six stages referred to as the *trans theoretical model of behavior change*: precontemplation, contemplation, preparation, action, maintenance, and termination. During the precontemplation stage, individuals are not really thinking about making any changes, do not see their behavior as problematic, and are typically not ready for change. When individuals are in the contemplation stage, they recognize there is a problem, are thinking about making a change, and usually getting ready to make change. During the preparation stage, individuals are ready to make a change and may actually begin making small changes in their behavior. During the action phase, individuals are making consistent apparent changes in their behavior. In the maintenance stage, individuals have made changes for a sustained period, usually 6 months or longer, and are working to prevent any setbacks. During the final stage of change – termination – individuals have sustained the maintenance stage for quite some time and have no desire to return to their previous behaviors. Coaches and trainers need to be aware of these stages of change when working with individuals who need to change their behaviors as a result of disordered eating.

Ergogenic Aids and Dietary Supplements

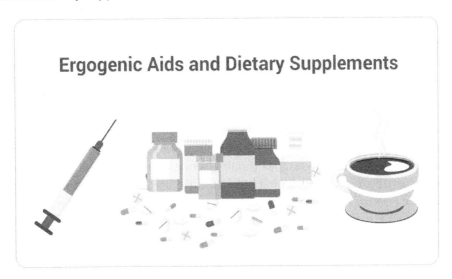

There are a variety of ergogenic aids and dietary supplements on the market available to athletes, and the options continue to grow as more supplements are created. Ergogenic aids are considered to be any substance, device, or practice that has the ability to enhance or improve an individual's performance. They can be categorized as nutritional, pharmacologic, physiologic, or psychologic substances. Availability and use of ergogenic aids have increased tremendously in the last 10 years, and research indicates that about half of the general population, 76% of college athletes, and nearly all athletes engaged in strength building use ergogenic aids. Some popular ergogenic aids for increasing muscle mass and strength include creatine, beta-hydroxyl beta-methylbuteric acid (HMB), protein and amino acids, and beta-alanine. Popular aerobic endurance nutrition supplements include branched-chain amino acids (BCAAs), caffeine, sodium tablets, glutamine, high molecular weight carbohydrates, protein, sodium bicarbonate and citrate, and sports beverages.

Ergogenic aids for increasing muscle mass and strength
Creatine
Creatine is a naturally occurring substance that is found in the kidneys, liver, and pancreas. It consists of the amino acids glycine, arginine, and methionine and can be found in protein sources such as meat and

fish. Creatine supplementation is used to improve strength, increase lean body mass, and potentially aid rapid muscle recovery during exercise. Creatine converts to creatine phosphate in the body, which is needed to make ATP, the energy molecule for muscle contractions. While research indicates that creatine can improve performance in high-intensity exercise, evidence does not support its use in endurance sports because it does not appear to affect aerobic metabolism. Creatine monophosphate supplements are considered to be safe if used in recommended amounts by healthy individuals. The ISSN position on creatine monophosphate supplements concludes that creatine is an effective ergogenic nutrition supplement in athletes to enhance high-intensity exercise and lean body mass. The recommended regimen by the ISSN to increase muscle creatine is to take 0.3 grams per kilogram of body weight per day of creatine monohydrate for at least 3 days, then 3-5 grams per day to maintain the increased stores. Creatine at the rate of about 0.1 grams per kilogram of body weight per day added to a protein supplement may help further facilitate resistance training. The ISSN concludes that creatine monophosphate supplements may be used in youth athletes under proper guidance and supervision.

Beta Hydroxyl Beta-Methylbuteric Acid
Beta hydroxyl beta-methylbuteric acid (HMB) comes from the amino acid leucine. HMB plays a role in the prevention of protein breakdown, or proteolysis. As a result, it is used in individuals with muscle wasting conditions and by athletes to enhance performance. HMB may be useful for individuals who are starting a strength training program and seeking to increase lean body mass. HMB can be safely used by youth and adults. Although HMB is commonly used as a supplement, it can be found in citrus fruits, catfish, and milk.

Protein and Amino Acids
Protein is needed for muscle atrophy during strength training. The body needs to remain in positive nitrogen balance to prevent muscle atrophy and catabolism, which is the breakdown of muscle that occurs when protein is inadequate. Resistance training, along with positive nitrogen balance, is needed to build muscle. As such, protein or its building blocks (amino acids) must be present to ensure positive nitrogen balance. The RDA for protein of 0.8 grams per kilogram of body weight may be sufficient as a minimum for individuals not engaged in strength training; however, individuals engaged in strength training require at least 1.2-1.7 grams per kilogram of body weight.

When considering protein intake, it is also important to consider the type of protein—complete or incomplete. Complete proteins contain all of the EAAs and usually come from animal sources. Incomplete proteins contain some of the essential nutrients and are found in foods such as beans, nuts, seeds, and grains. Incomplete proteins can be combined with other incomplete proteins or complete proteins to provide a complete amino acid profile. Athletes may also use other sources of protein isolates such as whey, casein, or soy in the form of powders, bars, drinks, etc.

Beta-alanine
Beta-alanine is used to enhance athletic performance, particularly high-intensity, anaerobic activities. Beta-alanine, a non-EAA, is a component of carnosine, along with histidine, and is produced in skeletal muscle. Carnosine is an essential buffering element in skeletal muscle. If beta-alanine is not present, carnosine production cannot occur. Beta-alanine supplementation increases muscle carnosine content, which helps to improve performance during high-intensity exercise by neutralizing acid production. Beta-alanine is usually supplemented in amounts of 3-6 grams per day for athletes engaged in anaerobic activity who are seeking performance enhancement.

Ergogenic Aids for Increasing Aerobic Endurance

Branched-Chain Amino Acids

Branched-chain amino acids (BCAAs), sometimes called the *proteinogenic amino acids,* are essential nutrients for building protein and include leucine, isoleucine, and valine. The term *branched-chain* refers to the chemical structure of the nutrients. BCAA usage is becoming increasingly popular with athletes engaged in aerobic activity, as they are believed to enhance recovery from exercise, reduce muscle damage, and decrease central fatigue. Research studies have used a range of doses for BCAAs; however, the optimal dose is not clear. Dosing for BCAAs should be based on body weight and intensity and duration of exercise.

Caffeine

Caffeine is the most widely used stimulant in the world. Research on the use and potential benefits of caffeine and athletic performance has continued to evolve, but current prevailing studies indicate that caffeine enhances endurance and alertness and reduces muscle soreness. Caffeine is known to be a mild diuretic, and as such, can potentially lead to dehydration during exercise activity if consumed in large amounts; however, this problem has not been widely cited in the literature. The International Olympic Committee allows athletes to have up to 12 micrograms per milliliter of caffeine in their urine, and the National Collegiate Athletic Association (NCAA) allows 15 micrograms per milliliter in urine before any violation is cited. Optimal dosing of caffeine ranges from 3 to 6 milligrams per kilogram of body weight. Some individuals believe that caffeine should be eliminated from an athlete's diet prior to competition and that, because it is considered a gateway drug, youth should not be allowed to use caffeine.

Sodium Tablets

Sodium tablets for electrolyte replacement help prevent hyponatremia during exercise. The tablets usually contain sodium chloride, which is a dissolved salt in the body. Athletes who have hypertension or kidney disease should not take sodium supplements.

Glutamine

Glutamine, a nonessential and most abundant amino acid, is found in the blood and muscles. Dietary sources of glutamine include beef, pork, chicken, fish, eggs, and dairy products. It has been shown to be effective in preventing illness and infection and reducing or preventing muscle soreness.

High Molecular-Weight Carbohydrates

High molecular-weight carbohydrates help athletes by replenishing glycogen stores and increasing gastric emptying, compared to other starches such as maltodextrin and dextrose. Waxy maize is an example of a high molecular-weight carbohydrate that does not contain sugar and is rapidly absorbed. Protein, as mentioned earlier, can be used in conjunction with carbohydrates to rebuild glycogen stores after exercise and has been shown to be more efficacious than high molecular-weight carbohydrates alone.

Sodium Bicarbonate

The use of sodium bicarbonate with caffeine 70-90 minutes before exercise has been shown to reduce fatigue. Sodium bicarbonate is essentially a buffer, which helps to prevent the acidic environment associated with fatigue during anaerobic activity. Sodium bicarbonate with citrate may lead to gastrointestinal discomfort, so it may not be the best solution for athletes.

Sports Beverages

Sports beverages support hydration, prevent hyponatremia through the maintenance and restoration of electrolytes, and help reduce fatigue during prolonged aerobic activity. Sports beverages can be divided into three categories: isotonic, hypertonic, and hypotonic. Isotonic beverages contain sodium and sugar in physiologically similar levels; hypertonic beverages contain more sodium and sugar than the body; and hypotonic beverages contain lower amounts of sodium and sugar than the body. Some believe that sports beverages with higher amounts of sodium and sugar are not needed unless athletes are engaged in activity lasting over 90 minutes. Sports beverages should ideally contain about 6%-8% carbohydrates and be ingested at a rate of 3-8 ounces every 10-20 minutes for activities lasting around 90 minutes or longer.

Signs and Symptoms of Ergogenic Aid Abuse

Since ergogenic aids can enhance athletic performance, there is potential of abuse. However, ergogenic aids can adversely affect major body systems including the cardiovascular, endocrine, genitourinary, dermatological, hepatic, musculoskeletal, and psychological systems. Signs and symptoms of ergogenic aid abuse include changes in blood lipids, increased blood pressure, and decreased myocardial function; gynecomastia (enlarged breasts), decreased sperm count, shrunken testicles, impotence, and infertility in men; menstrual irregularities, enlarged clitoris, deepened voice, and a more masculine appearance for women; acne and baldness; increased chance for liver tumors and damage; increased risk of tendon tears, intramuscular abscesses, and early epiphyseal plate closure; and depression, mood swings, hostility, and aggressive violent behavior.

Specific ergogenic aids banned by the Olympics and/or the NCAA include amphetamines, anabolic steroids, androstenediol, androstenedione, blood doping, dehydroepiandrosterone (DHEA), ephedrine, and human growth hormone. The Drug Enforcement Agency (DEA), the agency in the United States responsible for controlling the issues associated with controlled pharmaceuticals and chemicals, prohibits the sale or possession of anabolic steroids without the prescription of a physician. Violators may be subject to fines and/or imprisonment.

The World Anti-Doping Agency has a complete list of performance enhancement substances (PES) that are prohibited at their website (https://www.wada-ama.org/); the major categories of PES that are prohibited include anabolic agents; peptide hormones, growth factors, related substances, and mimetics; beta-2 antagonists; hormone and metabolic modulators; diuretics and masking agents; stimulants; narcotics; cannabinoids; and glucocorticoids.

Practice Questions

1. Which meal planning approach may be best suited for an individual seeking to lower blood pressure through weight loss?
    a. Healthy U.S. Eating Style
    b. Food exchanges
    c. DASH Eating Plan
    d. Glycemic index

2. What is the typical recommended carbohydrate intake for athletes?
    a. 3-7 grams of carbohydrate per kilogram of body weight
    b. 4-8 grams of carbohydrate per kilogram of body weight
    c. 5-9 grams of carbohydrate per kilogram of body weight
    d. 6-10 grams of carbohydrate per kilogram of body weight

3. An athlete would like to gain muscle mass. With regard to diet, what should the athlete be instructed to do?
    a. Supplement the diet with branched-chain amino acids.
    b. Consume protein in the diet in excess of needs to help build lean tissue.
    c. Eat a diet that consists of 1.5-2.0 grams per kilogram of body weight.
    d. Add protein powder to meals and snacks as needed.

4. Which of the following statements is most accurate about vitamin and mineral supplementation for athletes?
    a. Athletes cannot meet their nutrition needs with food alone.
    b. Most athletes require vitamin and mineral supplementation.
    c. Vitamin and mineral supplements help to improve athletic performance.
    d. Vitamin and mineral supplements can help to correct a deficiency.

5. Which statement best describes current advice about dietary and blood cholesterol?
    a. Cholesterol is produced in the body but also needed through some foods.
    b. Dietary cholesterol has little impact on blood cholesterol.
    c. Foods high in saturated fats do not typically contain cholesterol.
    d. A normal range for cholesterol is below 220 milligrams per deciliter.

6. Which athlete is at the highest risk for iron-deficiency anemia?
    a. Male athlete who strength trains regularly
    b. Female endurance athlete
    c. Adolescent athlete
    d. Female vegan athlete who strength trains

7. Dehydration at which level can negatively affect athletic performance?
    a. 1% of body weight
    b. 2% of body weight
    c. 3% of body weight
    d. 5% of body weight

8. Nutritional rating systems designed to help with selecting nutrient-dense foods include all EXCEPT which of the following?
   a. Glycemic index
   b. Nutripoints
   c. Food exchanges
   d. Points Food System

9. Which macronutrient composition is best suited for short-term weight loss?
   a. 70% carbohydrate, 20% protein, and 10% fat
   b. 60% carbohydrate, 20% protein, and 20% fat
   c. 55% carbohydrate, 30% protein, and 25% fat
   d. 45% carbohydrate, 30% protein, and 25% fat

10. Which statement best describes nutrient timing?
    a. Nutrient timing is altering the content of the total diet.
    b. Nutrient timing is altering the total content and timing of the total diet.
    c. Nutrient timing is altering the carbohydrate and protein content and timing of the diet.
    d. Nutrient timing is altering the carbohydrate and fat content and timing of the diet.

11. Carbohydrate loading is recommended for activities lasting longer than 100 minutes and can be accomplished by consuming which of the following?
    a. 8-10 grams of carbohydrate per kilogram of body weight
    b. 7-9 grams of carbohydrate per kilogram of body weight
    c. 6-8 grams of carbohydrate per kilogram of body weight
    d. 5-7 grams of carbohydrate per kilogram of body weight

12. Essential amino acids are required by the body and include which of the following?
    a. Arginine and cysteine
    b. Isoleucine and lysine
    c. Alanine and glycine
    d. Glutamine and histidine

13. Which of the following is most correct regarding eating disorders?
    a. Eating disorders are not attributed to genetics.
    b. Eating disorders can be resolved in a matter of months.
    c. Eating disorders align with a set of specific criteria.
    d. Eating disorders are usually attributed to stress.

14. A coach notices that an athlete seems to have a distorted body image, and the athlete reports using laxatives to cleanse the body. This behavior aligns with what eating disorder?
    a. Anorexia nervosa
    b. Bulimia nervosa
    c. Binge eating disorder
    d. An unspecified eating disorder

15. Which of the following statements is accurate about ergogenic aids?
    a. About 30% of the general population use ergogenic aids.
    b. The use of ergogenic aids is decreasing.
    c. About 76% of college athletes use ergogenic aids.
    d. Ergogenic aids are substances that enhance an individual's performance.

16. An athlete would like to start using creatine as an ergogenic aid. The athlete should receive which of the following advice?
    a. Creatine can be made in the body and supplementation is not safe for athletes.
    b. Research indicates that creatine is best suited for endurance sports.
    c. The ISSN has concluded that athletes should consider other ergogenic aids.
    d. Creatine can be started at 0.3 grams per kilogram of body weight.

17. Beta hydroxyl beta-methylbuteric acid (HMB) plays a role in the prevention of what?
    a. Cytolysis
    b. Hydrolysis
    c. Proteolysis
    d. Hydrogenolysis

18. Which amino acid must be present for the development of carnosine, an essential muscle buffering element?
    a. Histidine
    b. Beta-alanine
    c. Carnosine
    d. Leucine

19. An athlete would like to use an ergogenic aid for delaying fatigue. Which of the following is a good option?
    a. Sodium tablets and/or sports beverages
    b. Glutamine and/or sodium tablets
    c. Branched-chain amino acids and/or caffeine
    d. Sports beverages and/or caffeine

20. Which of the following is an example of a high molecular-weight carbohydrate?
    a. Sodium bicarbonate
    b. Maltodextrin
    c. Dextrose
    d. Waxy maize

21. Which of the following is a banned ergogenic aid?
    a. Amphetamines
    b. Insulin
    c. Glucose tablets
    d. Hydroxycut

Answer Explanations

1. C: The DASH Eating Plan is based on clinical research trials, which helped individuals lower their blood pressure and low-density lipoprotein (LDL) cholesterol and improve heart health. The Healthy U.S. Eating Style, food exchanges, and glycemic index are not specifically designed to help individuals lower their blood pressure.

2. D: Carbohydrate needs for athletes vary depending on the intensity, duration, and frequency of exercise, but typically range from 6 to 10 grams of carbohydrate per kilogram of body weight. The amounts given in other answer choices might supply nonathletic individuals with sufficient carbohydrate intake, but research indicates that athletes need 6-10 grams per kilogram of body weight.

3. C: Protein requirements vary depending on the type, duration, and frequency of exercise, but recommendations usually range from 1.5 to 2.0 grams per kilogram of body weight per day for athletes. Supplementing the diet with branched-chain amino acids can supply additional protein, but the focus should be on dietary sources through whole foods. Excessive protein is converted and stored as fat and does not contribute to increased lean body mass.

4. D: Vitamin and mineral supplementation does not improve athletic performance but can help to correct a deficiency if one is present. Athletes can usually meet their nutritional requirements with food, and therefore, supplementation is not typically necessary.

5. B: High cholesterol is a risk factor for heart disease, but research indicate that dietary cholesterol does not significantly impact blood cholesterol. Cholesterol is required by the body for various physiological and structural functions. However, these requirements are met by the cholesterol produced in the body; little to no additional cholesterol is needed from the diet. Foods high in saturated fat also typically contain cholesterol. A normal range for cholesterol is 200 milligrams per deciliter or lower, not 220 milligrams per deciliter.

6. D: Of the given choices, a female vegan athlete would be at the highest risk for iron-deficiency anemia. Iron recommendations are 1.3-1.7 times higher for athletes than nonathletes in general and another 1.8 times higher for vegetarian athletes in comparison to those who eat animal protein. While females and adolescents are at high risk for iron-deficiency anemia, a female vegan athlete would be at a higher risk.

7. B: Decreased physical performance can occur when dehydration levels cause a reduction in just 2% of body weight.

8. C: The food exchange system is designed to support meal planning but not necessarily the selection of nutrient-dense foods. The other options are all systems designed to be used in nutritional profiling or rating to support selecting nutrient-dense foods.

9. D: Macronutrient composition needs to be tailored to the individual based on body composition, training, and goals, but a caloric distribution of about 40%-45% carbohydrate, 30%-35% protein, and 25% fat should lead to body fat loss in the short term. The other options all provide a higher amount of carbohydrate than would be optimal for short-term weight loss.

10. C: Nutrient timing refers to effectively altering the content of the diet, particularly carbohydrate and protein, combined with the right timing to deliver optimal health and performance. Nutrient timing does not refer to altering the total content of the diet, the total content of the diet and timing, or the carbohydrate, fat, and timing of the diet.

11. A: Carbohydrate loading is typically recommended for activities lasting longer than 120 minutes by consuming a high-carbohydrate diet of about 8-10 grams of carbohydrate per kilogram of body weight. The ranges listed for carbohydrate loading in the other options are not supported by research.

12. B: This option has the correct combination of essential amino acids, while the other options include conditional and/or nonessential amino acids. Arginine and cysteine are conditional amino acids; alanine and glycine are nonessential amino acids; and glutamine and histidine are conditional amino acids.

13. C: This option is correct, since the other statements about eating disorders are not accurate. An eating disorder is a diagnosed mental illness with a specific set of eating patterns and behaviors as described in the *Diagnostic and Statistical Manual of Mental Disorders* (DSM) published by the American Psychiatric Association. Eating disorders are attributed to genetics, cannot be resolved in a matter of months, and are not attributed to stress.

14. B: In bulimia nervosa (BN), similar to anorexia nervosa (AN), individuals typically have distorted body image. Individuals with AN have a distorted body image but do not engage in purging behaviors. Binge eating disorder is closely related to BN, but individuals do not engage in purging or other compensatory behaviors to eliminate consumed foods. An unspecified eating disorder is one that does not align specifically with the criteria for the AN, BN, or binge eating disorder.

15. C: About 76% of college athletes and nearly all athletes engaged in strength building exercise use ergogenic aids. Ergogenic aids are used by about half of the general population, and research indicates their use has increased in the last 10 years. Ergogenic aids not only enhance athletic performance, but also include nutritional, pharmacologic, physiologic, or psychologic substances.

16. D: A recommended regimen by the ISSN to increase muscle creatine is to start taking 0.3 grams per kilogram of body weight per day of creatine monohydrate for at least 3 days. Creatine is a naturally occurring substance that is found in the kidneys, liver, and pancreas, and the ISSN states that it can be safely and effectively used to enhance high-intensity exercise and lean body mass. Evidence does not support the use of creatine in endurance sports because it does not appear to have an effect on aerobic metabolism.

17. C: Beta hydroxyl beta-methylbuteric acid (HMB) plays a role in the prevention of protein breakdown, or proteolysis. HMB does not play a role in cytolysis, hydrolysis, or hydrogenolysis.

18. B: Beta-alanine is the specific nonessential amino acid that must be present for the development of carnosine. Histidine is a component of carnosine; carnosine and leucine are not required for the development of carnosine.

19. C: Branched-chain amino acids and caffeine is the best answer choice, since the other options do not represent combinations of ergogenic aids that are used to delay fatigue. Sodium tablets help to prevent hyponatremia during exercise. Glutamine is used typically to help prevent illness and infection and reduce or prevent muscle soreness. Sports beverages are used for hydration and the prevention of hyponatremia and fatigue; however, caffeine is used as a stimulant to enhance endurance, increase alertness, and improve muscle soreness.

20. D: Waxy maize is the correct choice, since the other options are not considered to be high molecular weight carbohydrates. Sodium bicarbonate is used in combination with caffeine to help reduce fatigue. Maltodextrin and dextrose are starches but not considered to be high molecular weight.

21. A: Amphetamines are correct because the other options are permitted in sports. Insulin, glucose tablets, and Hydroxycut are not substances that are classified as ergogenic aids and, thus, are not banned.

Exercise Technique

Resistance Training Exercise Technique

Chronic resistance training affords strength, power, and coordination improvements, as well as greater efficiency of the anaerobic systems. Nervous system adaptations occur quickly with training as motor units (an alpha motor neuron from the spinal cord and all of the skeletal muscle fibers it supplies) become conditioned to activate more efficiently, more quickly, and more often. These adaptions increase the neural stimulation for muscle fibers to contract. As more motor units activate and coordinate with each other, a higher percentage of fibers in a muscle contract simultaneously, which increases contractile strength. In fact, many of the earliest strength improvements noticed in resistance training programs are due to these neural adaptations, rather than muscle hypertrophy (which takes approximately 4-8 weeks to occur). An athlete can quickly experience increases in strength and power as a result of training. Over time, muscle fibers increase in size while bone mineral density increases in load-bearing bones, helping mitigate age-related bone and muscle loss.

Free Weight Training Equipment
Dumbbells and barbells are the most commonly used free weight training equipment. While both involve "lifting weights," this equipment differs from resistance machines in that weight plates, dumbbells, and barbells are used in varying weights for any number of exercises being typically held in the hands of the athlete. Conversely, machines are prearranged setups where the athlete simply adjusts the weight and machine height. With machine equipment, an athlete can typically perform a minimal number of designated movements per machine, which are specifically designed for that exercise.

Preparatory Body and Limb Position
Proper form, including position and stance, varies depending on the free weight exercise. There are also modifications of basic exercises that alter grip position as a way to provide a different challenge to the muscles and stress particular fibers. For example, typical dumbbell curls can occur in a standing or seated position, depending on the workout and goal of the exercise. The standing position recruits additional muscles, such as those in the core, to stabilize the body. When the exercise is done in a seated position, core muscles do not need to work as hard because the body's weight is supported by the chair, but this modification does require the targeted muscles (in this case, the biceps) to be more isolated and consequently work harder to lift the weight unassisted by any momentum that may be gathered while standing and swaying the body. Even with very skilled and disciplined athletes, the weight lifted during a seated curl may be less than standing due to this muscle isolation. Therefore, trainers must consider the trade-offs of the two positions: adding a core workout component to a standing exercise versus truly isolating the primary muscle more directly by sitting. Whether standing or sitting, athletes should be mindful to maintain proper posture with an erect spine, the shoulders back, chest out, and eyes gazing straight forward. Feet should be shoulder-width or slightly wider apart, and knees should have a slight bend when standing. During a seated curl, feet should be positioned flat on the floor under the knees, which are flexed to 90 degrees.

- *Grips*: As mentioned, grip position can also be tweaked. In a standard biceps curl, the athlete holds the dumbbell in the middle of the bar with a *supinated grip*, allowing muscle fibers to work equally and in the typical sagittal plane of motion for flexion. In a variation called *hammer curls*, the athlete holds the dumbbell in the middle of the bar but with a 90-degree internal rotation of the wrist so that palms are facing the hips, which is called a *neutral grip*. This places slightly more of the workload on the lateral fibers of the biceps, working the lateral head more than the standard grip position. *Pronated grip* is also called *overhand grip* and occurs when the palms face the floor and the knuckles face the ceiling. In contrast, the supinated grip is also called *underhand grip* and palms face up while knuckles face the floor. *Alternated grip* is when one hand is pronated and the other is supinated; *closed grip* is when the thumb is wrapped around the bar; and *false grip* is when the thumb does not wrap around the bar. Another grip pattern is called *hook grip* and it is similar to a pronated grip except that the thumb is moved under the index and middle fingers.

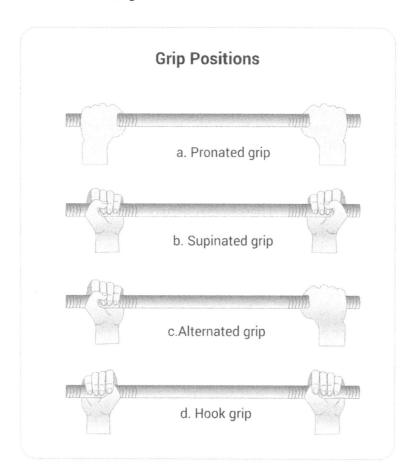

- *Squats*: Feet are typically slightly further than shoulder-width apart, and toes should be pointing straight forward. As the athlete lowers the body into the squatted position, the hips should go backwards as if they are reaching to sit back in a chair, and the flexed knees should not come forward beyond the toes. Athletes should visualize pushing up through their heels to return to the fully upright position. Before performing squats, when facing the bar, it should be racked prior to execution at mid- to upper-chest level.

- *Free Weight Exercises*: Significantly more focus should be placed on proper form and stability of the body than resistance machines, which typically support the body in the correct position and only allow movement in the desired plane. Because of this, particularly in less experienced athletes, the weight lifted in free weight exercises may be lower for any given exercise than that successfully attempted with the equivalent resistance machine. Strength coaches should pay attention to lifting form to ensure that athletes are not swinging the weights, attempting to lift weights that are too heavy and relying on momentum for assistance, or using improper form, all which can increase injury risk.

Execution of Technique
The proper execution of lifting exercises with free weights should be demonstrated and explained thoroughly by strength coaches. Athletes often have different learning styles, so the execution and explanation of proper form and technique in exercises is imperative to convey this information to each athlete. Each exercise obviously has its own set of procedures for proper execution, but in general, emphasis on form and breathing technique will lead to successful execution. With exercises that are completed in a standing position, knees should be slightly relaxed and not locked, feet should be facing forward, and a strong core should be engaged to support the erect spine. Exercises in the seated and supine positions require five points of contact for optimal body support: the head is firmly on the bench or back pad, the shoulders and upper back are evenly placed and firmly on the bench or back pad, the buttocks are positioned evenly on the bench or seat, and the right and left foot are both placed flat on the floor.

In American society today, daily activities tend to focus on forward posture such as typing on a computer or holding a cell phone in front of the face and hunching over to type on it. This chronic slouched posture can lead to tightness in the anterior muscles of the chest and a stretching and weakening of posterior muscles of the shoulders, neck, and upper back. Strength coaches often need to remind athletes to pull their shoulders back and engage their rhomboids and keep their chest up and out, which opens it up for both improved breathing mechanics and a healthy posture. In all standing exercises, swinging the weights should be avoided, and athletes should attempt to hold their bodies as still in the upright position as possible, refraining from swaying and rocking, which uses momentum to augment the lifting motion. Athletes should be instructed to exhale, mostly through the mouth, during the concentric or more challenging lifting portion of the movement through the sticking point (the hardest point of the exercise). They should then inhale slowly through the nose during the eccentric or easier phase, depending on the motion. In most cases, holding the breath such as in the Valsalva maneuver is contraindicated, and it can greatly increase blood pressure and cause dizziness and disorientation. However, it can be used in certain core exercises with care as a way to increase torso rigidity and aid support of the vertebral column. This lessens compressive forces on the intervertebral discs and supports the normal and neutral lordotic lumbar spine. These same benefits can be achieved through the use of a weight belt, which should be used for exercises that stress the lower back, especially at near maximal loads.

With the exception of power exercises, free weight exercises should use a minimum of one or two spotters when an athlete moves the bar over the head or face, has it on the front of the shoulders, or positioned on the back during the execution. When performing an incline bench press, the weight bar should make contact with the upper chest at the sticking point. In contrast, with a flat or decline bench press, the bar should make contact slightly lower – at or below nipple line. There are a variety of squats depending on the location of the bar, including front squats, back squats, and split squats (sort of like a stationary lunge). With deadlifts, the conventional lift has feet spaced about hip-width apart and hands outside of the stance. The sumo modification places the feet wider than a conventional squat, outside of shoulder-width, and hands are inside of the stance. Romanian deadlifts are similar to conventional ones in that feet are hip-width and hands are outside of the stance.

- *Common Mistakes*: Athletes should only lift the weight that they are able to manage while safely completing the exercise with proper form through the entire range of motion, maintaining control of the weight during the lowering, eccentric phase. A common mistake is selecting a weight that is too heavy for the athlete, so it cannot be lifted through the full range, and then is dropped quickly when being lowered with gravity in a hurried, uncontrolled manner. For example, if an athlete is doing a dumbbell chest press, the weights should be pushed all the way up until the elbows are straight (but not locked), with the arms fully extended up and away from the chest. If the weight is too heavy, the athlete cannot fully extend the arms and noticeable flexion will remain in the elbows. As the weights are brought back down to either side of the chest, the coach may notice the weights plummet precipitously and may even drop to the floor. This is not only dangerous, but negates the muscular work of slowly lowering the weight, so the athlete misses out on this training effect and strength benefit.

- *Arousal*: For maximal benefit from any resistance exercise, athletes should dedicate their focus on form and breathing, concentrating on the workout, keeping distracting conversations to a minimum. There is an optimal point on the arousal-relaxation curve, also known as the "Inverted U" due to its shape, for best performance — somewhere in the middle of the two extremes of being too lackadaisical and too anxious about the lift. Some anticipation, anxiety, and arousal leads to increased levels of epinephrine, which actually primes the system for increased strength performance. On the other hand, too much stress and arousal can flood the system with epinephrine and increase heart rate and blood pressure beyond helpful levels. This can lead to a detrimental state where the exercise on top of the increased sympathetic nervous system response drives these physiologic variables too high, resulting in the body reducing its physical output during the exercise. These athletes may need coaches to calm them, working on relaxing visualizations, and working to reduce pressure to lower their arousal state so that excess epinephrine does not negatively impact performance. An athlete that is too relaxed and unfocused does not reap the benefit of this hormonal influence on performance, and these athletes may need cheering, motivation, verbal "pumping up," and some small stimulus of external pressure to increase their arousal.

Correction of Improper Technique
Strength coaches must correct improper technique as early as possible in the learning process to prevent the development of bad habits and to reduce the risk of injury. Even advanced athletes may demonstrate poor technique when fatigued, distracted, or unmotivated, so observing and giving cues on

preparatory and execution form techniques need to be a constant focus of strength coaches during workouts. For maximal effectiveness, feedback should be as specific and timely as possible, and should be visual, auditory, and kinesthetic, depending on each athlete's learning style. Strength coaches may position athletes in front of the mirror so they can observe and self-correct deviations in form, sometimes concurrent with a proper form demonstration alongside the athlete for comparison. Coaches can also pair up athletes with differing skill levels to promote a learning/teaching mentorship. This can also help more experienced athletes develop leadership roles while also finding a reason to focus on their own form, which may need some fine-tuning as the athlete becomes complacent with experience. Strength coaches can use videos and handouts to also supplement learning or break down exercises into smaller movement steps for kinesthetic learners. Regardless of the delivery method, all form correction feedback should be positive, supportive, and instructive to foster a warm learning environment and keep the athlete motivated and comfortable.

Resistance Machines

Resistance machines typically enable the proper form to be achieved more easily for exercises because they only allow movement in certain planes of motion based on the mechanical setup of the levers, hinges, pulleys, and movable pieces. However, this guidance, restriction, and stabilization make exercises completed on resistance machines less sports-specific than free weights, plyometric, or body weight exercises in which the athlete must stabilize the body while moving through the range of motion. Weight machines can be a good starting place for beginners and also for senior athletes and others who have poor balance and coordination, and for certain exercises for individuals recovering from injuries. This is because these machines are generally safer to use and usually only isolate one movement, which makes them easier to use and a good way for beginners to grasp one specific movement at a time. Resistance machines can be helpful for rehabilitating certain body parts because they generally isolate a specific muscle group. In general, this is not advantageous for overall strength-training, especially for sports-specific work important to competitive athletes. However, resistance machines have their place, particularly in injury rehab, solo sessions, rapid circuit training, and reaching higher maximal lifts. For heavy weights and maximal efforts, most machines have the advantage of not requiring a spotter, although athletes should still always exercise caution when attempting any lift. Some machines force the correct movement for the lift, which may help reduce the risk of injury and ensure that the athlete is moving through the entire range of motion for each repetition. Machine workouts can be more efficient because they are generally organized in a circuit in the layout of the gym, so the athlete can easily move from one to another. With that said, if athletes prioritize saving time and they do not properly adjust the settings to fit the machine to their body, athletes can "cheat" in the movement and increase injury risk.

As mentioned previously, most weight machines require the athlete to move the weight in a predetermined path, making it difficult to strengthen the stabilizer muscles. Similarly, usually only one exercise can be completed on each machine, making it cumbersome to keep getting up, moving to another machine, and adjusting the settings accordingly. Most machines are designed for the average-sized adult, so small youth athletes, slight women, or significantly taller and larger athletes may find the fit less than ideal, even when adjusted as much as possible, resulting in a fit that is not only uncomfortable, but may cause difficulty performing the exercise correctly.

Preparatory Body and Limb Position

Proper form with a good neutral erect spine, chest up and out, feet flat on the floor, and shoulders back should be used on machines. The height of the bench or chair portion can usually be adjusted and should be so that the knees are flexed to 90 degrees and the feet are flat on the floor. For machines such as the leg press, the feet should be placed on the platform slightly wider than hip-width. Knees should flex in alignment with the ankles, refraining from any tendency to deviate them laterally, which internally rotates the hips and places undo stress on the lateral compartment of the knee. Hand grip should be neutral and evenly spaced in most cases, unless a narrow or wide grip is specifically introduced as a modification. Most machines have pictures of proper alignment and positioning of pads and bars so that athletes can adjust the machine to fit their bodies. Athletes should align their joint axes with the axis of rotation of the machine to optimize joint function and prevent any incongruity in the moving axes, which can induce injury.

Execution of Technique
As with free weight exercises, proper technique on resistance machines is imperative, both to prevent injury and to maximize the benefit of the exercise. The proper execution of lifting exercises with free weights should be demonstrated and explained thoroughly by strength coaches. Each exercise obviously has its own set of procedures to carry it out properly, but in general, emphasis on form and breathing technique will lead to successful execution. Many resistance machines execute the movement in the seated position. As mentioned, exercises in the seated and supine positions require five points of contact for optimal body support: the head is firmly on the bench or back pad, the shoulders and upper back are evenly placed and firmly on the bench or back pad, the buttocks are positioned evenly on the bench or seat, and the right and left foot are both placed flat on the floor. The same general guidelines for execution that have been previously discussed should be employed with machine-based exercises as well.

Correction of Improper Technique
One of the benefits of resistance machines is that they make it more challenging to have improper technique compared to free weights and alternative strength-training modalities because of the constraints imposed by the design of the machines. Nevertheless, strength coaches should monitor athletes on the training floor and quickly correct any deviations from optimal form to prevent injury and to maximize training benefit. Athletes should be instructed to adjust settings on the machine, both in terms of sizing and resistance, to meet their individual bodies, even if working with a partner in a circuit when it would be more time-efficient to share the same setup. Mirrors work well to provide visual feedback to athletes, but their effectiveness is limited by the athlete's understanding of proper form, attention to detail, and the desire to perform exercises correctly. For this reason, strength coaches still need to heed attention to athletes using resistance machines.

Alternative Modes of Training
Alternative modes of training include core work, stability, balance, calisthenics, and bodyweight exercises. Such exercises augment training and may help prevent injuries. Plyometric training such as pull-ups, push-ups, chin-ups, squat thrusts, lunges, yoga, jumping jacks, and planks provide resistance in the form of bodyweight, so they improve relative strength and core strength, are low-cost, and improve body control. Many of these activities can be performed outside on the field or in an open gym with an entire team. Some coaches find that adding body work such as yoga to an athlete's regime improves flexibility, focus, breathing, core strength, and supports athletic goals in a less intense fashion. Strength coaches should educate athletes unfamiliar with these practices on their benefits to help improve acceptance and adherence. Calisthenics can be used in conjunction with dynamic warm-ups to prepare the athletes for practice and competition.

Preparatory Body and Limb Position
For push-ups and pull-ups, arms should be roughly shoulder-width apart, although modifications affecting hand spacing are often introduced to provide variable challenges to the muscles. For example, diamond push-ups have the athlete place his or her hands together, directly under the chest, with the index fingers and thumbs of each hand touching to form a diamond. This modification places extra

emphasis on the triceps, compared with the chest muscles such as the pectoralis major that are emphasized during a regular push-up. With core exercises, it is important that the spine stay neutral and that athletes do not pull up on their neck while doing crunches or sit-ups. They should use their core muscles to lift shoulder the blades off of the surface, with their hands simply supporting the weight of the head, but not pulling it upward. Yoga and Pilates incorporate many poses and positions and should be guided by a trained and certified professional. Lunges and squats require an athletic stance, feet slightly wider than hip-width apart and flat on the floor. For athletes who are limited in squat depth due to tight Achilles tendons, elevating the heels on a weight plate or other incline will help achieve a deeper squat, despite limited range of motion in the ankles. These athletes should be guided through a regular static stretching routine to help improve ankle mobility.

Execution of Technique
Bodyweight exercises improve relative, but not absolute, strength. With these exercises, athletes are often able to safely complete a higher number of repetitions than more traditional "weight lifting" exercises. This can improve muscular endurance and help prevent fatigue during long-duration activities. Athletes should inhale during the concentric or challenging phase through the sticking point and exhale on the eccentric or easier phase. The spine should stay neutral, with shoulders, hips, and ankles in alignment. While risk of injury is often lower with bodyweight-only exercises due to smaller loads than those imposed by external weights, proper form should still be followed.

Correction of Improper Technique
Strength coaches should pay close attention to athletes' form and technique for common mistakes such as a swayed back on push-ups or planks or raised buttocks above the plane of the body. Other issues to note include athletes using momentum during core work or craning and pulling the neck, and knees coming over the ankles with hips not sitting far enough back during squats and lunges. Because of the lack of external weights used during bodyweight exercises, it is sometimes easier to perform them with improper form without the athlete receiving any obvious physical signs of discomfort that are commonly experienced with weighted exercises. As with other forms of exercise, strength coaches must correct improper technique as early as possible in the learning process to prevent the development of bad habits as well as to reduce risk of injury. Even advanced athletes may demonstrate poor technique when fatigued, distracted, or unmotivated, so observing and giving cues on preparatory and execution form and technique should be the constant focus of strength coaches.

Non-Traditional Implements
In recent years, there has been an increased interest by athletes and coaches to implement non-traditional equipment for strength and resistance training, power and speed training, and overall conditioning. Tires, logs, water-filled pipes, sandbags, kettle bells, heavy battle ropes, and a variety of medicine balls have entered the training arena, popularized by some adventure races, CrossFit, and other innovative or rogue training programs. Such implements are creative ways to essentially add tools to the tool bag of a strength coach, while accomplishing similar physiologic goals for the athletes. Still, coaches must be aware of when and how to properly use this equipment and be sure to educate and supervise athletes in their use. Much of the non-traditional equipment is best reserved for advanced athletes who have the basic foundations of movements, such as a well-mastered squat and deadlift, because programs with non-traditional equipment tend to use heavier implements in power movements that can induce injury if not performed properly.

Preparatory Body and Limb Position
Some non-traditional training implements can be used to improve grip strength. Heavy ropes require the athlete to grip very tightly while forcefully swinging the ropes. Similarly, some sandbags lack

traditional handgrips, so the athlete must squeeze the material tightly while powerfully moving it. An athlete's stance and core engagement should be emphasized for all training exercises. For tire-flipping activities, athletes should use a wide base of support when squatting and keep the spine in the neutral lumbar lordosis position to protect the lower back and knees. A weight belt can help support the lumbar spine. Kettlebells offer somewhat of an exception to the rule against swinging weights and harnessing momentum, and in fact, many exercises specific to kettlebells rely on swinging for proper form, such as kettlebell swings. In this exercise, power should come from thrusting the hips forward and not from the shoulders lifting the implement.

Execution of Technique
Many of the non-traditional exercise tools provide a challenge for anaerobic and strength-building workouts. Strength coaches should demonstrate the proper execution of each movement and should consider the use of mirrors so that athletes can monitor their own form. Weight belts can be helpful in certain cases with maximal loads. As with traditional resistance exercises, athletes should exhale through the more challenging phase of the exercise, including the "sticking point," and then inhale slowly after the "sticking point" through the completion of the movement. The Valsalva maneuver is likely unavoidable with loads greater than 80% of maximal, but it does help stabilize the spine and decrease intradiscal pressure. When activities require speed, force, or a combination of the two (power), athletes should be prepped, focused, and ideally aroused to bring about optimal performance.

Correction of Improper Technique
Particularly when using a training implement for the first time, athletes will need extra supervision and critique of form. Strength coaches should be prudent to work with only a few athletes at a time so that athletes can get individualized attention, instruction, clarification if they have questions, and correction of improper form. While non-traditional equipment can bring fresh variety into a training program, it does have the potential for increased risk of injury if athletes are not properly trained, both in terms of their skill level as well as the particular instruction on the equipment usage.

Plyometric Exercise Technique

Plyometric training involves jumping and power exercises such as box jumps, squat thrusts, burpees, and hurdle drills to train the muscles to achieve maximal force in the shortest time. These explosive activities help strengthen an athlete's ligaments, tendons, joints, and muscles for sports-specific movements to better tolerate the physiologic demands of competition. Athletes who are susceptible to injury – particularly those with poor bone density, prior ligamentous or tendon injuries especially to the knees, or post-surgical individuals – should only do plyometric under carefully monitored and modified conditions due to the strains and forces induced by such explosive jumping. Young athletes and senior athletes can safely do plyometric training, but in a more modified fashion to control the load on the body. For example, box jumps or depth jumps are likely not safe for these populations, but bounding or skipping drills and one-legged hops can be implemented into programs in healthy athletes. However, the frequency of such activities should be limited to a day or two per week, with several rest days in-between. Even at such infrequent intervals, plyometrics can play a role in improving fitness and power without posing a substantial injury risk.

Preparatory Body and Limb Position
Plyometric exercises usually involve some sort of jumping, so athletes should be taught proper landing. This involves using the arms to reduce momentum and flexing the knees to attenuate the landing forces. Athletes should engage their core muscles to help brace the torso and to provide support to the intervertebral discs. It is imperative that athletes focus their eyes where they intend to jump to and

maintain mental focus during each individual repetition to prevent tripping and accidental injuries. It is best not to engage in such activities late in a workout when the neuromuscular system and mental focus might be fatigued. Most plyometrics are performed with either a relaxed hand or open and flat in the neutral position, with the palm facing the body, such as in sprinting form.

Execution of Technique

Plyometrics use quick, powerful movements that involve a pre-stretch or countermovement. This serves as a stretch-shortening cycle and increases the power of subsequent movements by harnessing the stretch reflex. It also uses the natural elastic components of tendons and muscles. With the stretch-shortening cycle, rapid eccentric contractions elicit the stretch reflex and the storage of elastic energy, which increases force production of the subsequent concentric contraction. Plyometrics can be completed for the lower body, trunk, and upper body areas and can include depth jumps, medicine ball throws, catches, pushups, box jumps, and bounding drills. Adequate rest is needed between repetitions (such as 5-10 seconds between box jumps) and 2-3 minutes between sets. Depending on the sport and skill level, these exercises should only be completed 1-3 times per week in training.

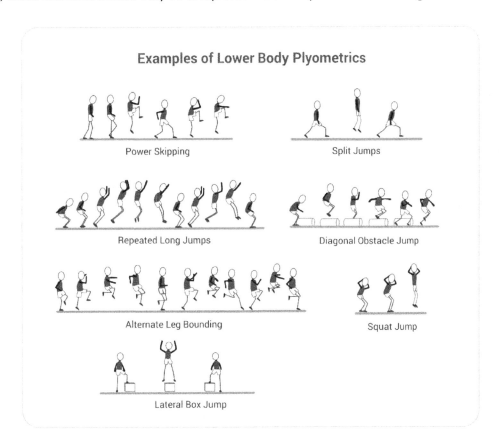

Examples of Lower Body Plyometrics

Power Skipping

Split Jumps

Repeated Long Jumps

Diagonal Obstacle Jump

Alternate Leg Bounding

Squat Jump

Lateral Box Jump

Correction of Improper Technique

Because of the demand on the body during plyometric exercises, proper technique is imperative to avoid injury. Also, heavier athletes (over 220 pounds) should be constantly monitored for any joint tenderness. Special care also must be considered for previously injured athletes, senior athletes, youth, and athletes with balance issues. Proper footwear and soft, rubberized flooring or grass should be used to reduce landing forces. With plyometrics, it is especially imperative that strength coaches correct improper technique as early as possible in the learning process to prevent the development of bad habits and to reduce the risk of injury. Even advanced athletes may demonstrate poor technique when fatigued, distracted, or unmotivated, so observing and giving cues on preparatory and execution form technique needs to be a constant focus. For maximal effectiveness, feedback should be as specific and timely as possible, and should be visual, auditory, and kinesthetic, depending on each athlete's learning style.

Teach and Evaluate Speed/Sprint Technique

Many athletes can benefit greatly from improving sprint and speed technique, which increases the maximal velocity with which they can accelerate and move. Strength, in the sense of sprinting, is somewhat different than with resistance training. Force application in sprinting enables the athlete to accelerate, reach high velocities, and maintain these speeds. Force is defined as mass multiplied by acceleration, and for athletic endeavors, rate of force development (RFD) combined with impulse are important, since force must be generated in a short time interval. Rate of force development is an index of explosive strength, referring to the development of maximal force in the minimal time interval, while impulse is the generated force multiplied by the time required for its production. Speed can be improved with sprint training, often resisted with sleds or parachutes, downhill and uphill training, and technical foot drills.

Fundamental training objectives for increasing running speed center on the following:

- Minimizing ground contact breaking forces: This can be accomplished by maximizing the backwards velocity of the foot and leg at touch-down and by working on creating this touch-down moment with the foot firmly under the center of gravity of the body.

- Emphasizing the brevity of ground support time: This helps bring about rapid stride rate, which takes explosive strength and can be improved through careful and specific plyometric exercise.

- Prioritizing functional training of the hamstring muscles: These muscles act simultaneously as concentric hip extensors and eccentric knee flexors: as the leg swings forward, the eccentric knee flexor strength has the greatest impact on the leg's recovery.

Preparatory Body and Limb Position
Track sprinters use blocks to help them accelerate rapidly by enabling a powerful push-off. These athletes essentially pre-load the leg like a spring, by pressing backwards onto the block with their flexed leg and dorsiflexed foot, storing potential energy in the series and elastic components of tendons and muscles. This enable a rapid transfer to kinetic energy when the race begins. The front knee is flexed about 90 degrees and the rear knee is flexed from 110-130 degrees. Hip angle varies with sprinting ability and experience. The front hip is flexed at 40 degrees in elite sprinters and 50 degrees in sub-elite sprinters. Additionally, the rear hip is at 80 degrees in elite sprinters and at 90 degrees in sub-elite sprinters. The athlete should place his or her hands just behind the starting line slightly wider than shoulder-width apart and the fingers held together. Each thumb should bridge out to the side and should be directly under each shoulder, ready to support the bodyweight. Gaze should be downward, with the back of the head and spine in a straight alignment.

Execution of Technique
Speed is influenced by stride rate and stride length, so athletes should focus on quick turnover and powerful steps. Of these factors, stride rate has a greater impact on speed and should be the focus when designing programs for improving sprinting speed. Elite sprinters are able to perform about 5 strides per second. As running speed approaches maximal for a given athlete, stride frequency increases more than stride length to contribute to additional speed gains. Ground contact time decreases about

50% from the acceleration phase to maximal velocity running. Impulse production becomes more and more dependent on the athlete's ability to generate explosive ground reaction forces (GRFs). The single leg support phase of running includes the eccentric braking component and the concentric propulsion. The flight phase of running is comprised of the recovery and ground preparation. Stride rate and stride length typically increase over the first 15-20 meters or 8-10 strides. During this time, forward lean decreases from about a 45-degree angle to fully upright by about 20 meters. Gaze should be directly forward, arms forcefully pumping at the sides with a lightly closed, relaxed fist or an open hand. Knees should drive upwards toward the chest. The core should be engaged to limit trunk rotation, support the diaphragm, and keep movement efficient. Arms should be flexed about 90 degrees and swing toward the forehead to help overcome inertia and to increase momentum. At the start of the sprint, runners push explosively out of the blocks. The rear leg produces the greater initial force but loses ground contact earlier. However, the front leg assumes a greater influence on starting velocity and exerts force for a longer duration. In elite athletes, the peak initial forces can exceed 1500 N and impulses can exceed 230 newton-seconds. In the final amount of extension in the front leg, the rear leg swings forward for the subsequent stride. During the acceleration stage, the swinging leg's thigh is perpendicular to the trunk and the lower leg is parallel to the trunk. At maximal velocity, the flexed leg acts like a pendulum and thrusts forward at the maximal speed to assist with leg power at push-off. The lower leg swings forward passively when the thigh reaches its maximal possible knee lift. When the forward leg starts to make contact with the ground at the toe, it makes light contact with the ground slightly in front of the body's center of gravity. As weight is transferred to this leg in the forward support phase of the body, the ball of the foot fully supports the body weight, and the trunk is fully upright or assumes a 5-degree forward lean. In the rear support phase, triple extension helps the body push up and propel forward in a hip-knee-ankle angle of 50-55 degrees, with propulsion velocity dependent on push-off impulse and direction. In the maximal velocity phase, leg drive ability is facilitated by explosive arm action, somewhat like hammering, where the hands swing forward above shoulder height and the upper arm is parallel to the trunk. Then the arm swings downward and backward past the pocket area and the hips. Shoulders should be held steady, elbows flexed to 90 degrees, and hands lightly cupped. The mouth should be left open and relaxed to prevent any unnecessary muscular fatigue.

Correction of Improper Technique

Coaches can help guide athletes to correct form and technique with drills such as high knees, bounding, turnover drills, resisted sprints, and assisted sprints (downhill). Video analyses and playback can be helpful as well as practicing with blocks. It can be difficult to truly change running form in a radical way, but speed can be improved significantly, along with aspects of technique through appropriate drills and a scientific approach to training. Parachutes and sled pulls provide added resistance to sprinting and strengthen the athlete's muscular and cardiovascular systems as well as force and power. However, they should be reserved for more trained and experienced athletes, particularly sled pulls, which can cause injury if form and technique are poor or if an athlete is fatigued, weak, prone to injury, pre-pubescent, or elderly. For children, parachutes are a safer choice but should still be used with caution. Deep water running and sprinting drills in shallow water can also be used to provide added resistance with the goal of improving strength, stamina, and ability.

Agility Technique

Agility is loosely defined as an athlete's collective coordinative abilities and technical skills used to perform the wide range of motor tasks of the sport from fine motor control to gross, powerful, and dynamic tasks. Agility is an important component of many athletic endeavors and relies on perceptual-cognitive ability as well as the ability to decelerate and re-accelerate in the intended directions and as quickly and seamlessly as possible. Combined with speed, agile athletes are able to outperform competitors with quicker ball-handling skills, breakaways, and tactics. Agility is not simply just about the change of directions, but involves changes in speed, decision-making, cognitive development, and biomechanical and metabolic efficiency. The following factors influence agility:

- Adaptive ability: how well the athlete can respond to observed and anticipated changes in the condition or sports situation and modify his or her actions accordingly
- Balance: the ability to establish and maintain static and dynamic equilibrium in the body
- Combinatory ability: ability to coordinate movements of the body during a given action
- Differentiation: the ability to accurately adjust body motions and mechanics in an efficient, economic way
- Orientation: body movements and control in terms of spatial and temporal parameters
- Reactiveness: the rapid, correct response to various stimuli
- Rhythm: ability to respond and implement appropriate timing and variation of dynamic motor patterns

These parameters vary in their degree of modifiability through training, depending on the athlete's age and skill level. Preadolescent athletes are generally in a time period considered to be critical and sensitive for skill development. During this time, the coordinative abilities are thought to be the most trainable. Training should center on more basic movement patterns to establish competency and build a strong baseline level of fitness. Younger athletes may not yet specialize in just one sport, which is actually advantageous for preventing injuries and developing a well-rounded athlete with the basic abilities needed for most athletic endeavors. During adolescence, athletes begin to lose some of this plasticity for skill development and should turn to specific skills and abilities for their targeted sport of focus. Agility training can include ladders, directional drills, cone drills, speed changes, line sprints, and other technique-driven footwork.

Preparatory Body and Limb Position
Preparatory body positioning for agility training depends on the exercise or drill to be performed. Nearly universally across exercises, athletes are standing with their gaze forward or slightly downward to keep targets in their peripheral vision. Arms should be relaxed in athletic position; hands have somewhat of a slight lateral angle that is deviated in some cases for additional balance; and bodyweight should be concentrated on the midfoot rather than the heel. This allows for quicker turnover and more precise movements. There is a tendency for the athlete to slouch or drop the shoulders downward while concentrating on the ground below the foot when using agility ladders, for example. However, it is important, as with all athletic activities, to attempt to maintain as much of an upright posture as possible, with a neutral spine and with the head and neck in alignment with the spine. Agility training requires tremendous visual and mental focus. Athletes should be reminded to breathe in a controlled and purposeful manner. Much of the training is not particularly demanding in a cardiovascular sense, but proper breathing mechanics are always important.

Execution of Technique
Agility training requires athletes to use quick, light steps so that they are able to change directions and speeds readily. Body weight should be concentrated on the forefoot, and knees should come up toward the chest by firing hip flexors and core muscles. Athletes should visualize the movement patterns prior to execution to strengthen the cognitive aspects of the agility training. For sports requiring a high degree

of agility, it's usually most effective to incorporate agility work on most days of an athletic training program, but only for a short time due to the technique and focus required.

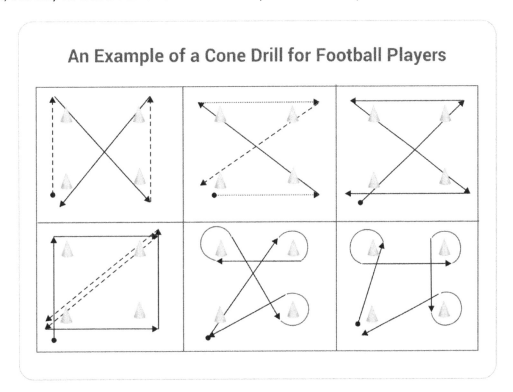

As an athlete fatigues, the completion time for various agility exercises will increase, both due to slower physical performance as well as reduced mental capacity, which causes increased reaction time and decision-making time. In almost all sports, agility and changes in direction or speed are not pre-planned or programmed, but must be made as instantaneous decisions. Athletes have to react to the environmental conditions, the game play, the movement and position of defending athletes, and ball position. Aspects of this on-the-fly decision-making ability are affected and improved simply with game experience over time, but some degree of rapid decision-making skills can be improved through agility drills.

Correction of Improper Technique
Strength coaches can use verbal cues and video analysis to help guide technique issues. Agility practice takes time and focus, and improvements can be slow. It is important for both the athlete and coach to set reasonable goals and be patient. A lack of agility for skills such as cornering, backward running, and certain maneuvers such as crossovers and sidestep cutting have been implicated as mechanisms of injury in athletes. Therefore, it is important that strength coaches take the time to work with athletes to improve agility, reaction time, coordinative abilities, and rhythm. As with all fitness modalities and aspects of training, strength coaches should correct improper technique as early as possible in the learning process and all form correction feedback should be positive, supportive, and instructive to foster a warm learning environment and keep the athlete motivated and comfortable.

Metabolic Conditioning/Energy Systems Development

Aerobic energy systems need to be trained for improvements in cardiovascular fitness, metabolic conditioning, and muscular endurance. These are important for all sports, and particularly so for endurance sports such as distance running, swimming, soccer, and cycling. Heart and skeletal muscle hypertrophy is one of the chronic adaptations with regular cardiovascular and resistance training, respectively. With cardiovascular training, as the heart enlarges and chamber size increases, allowing for a greater stroke volume and cardiac output. This also enables the heart to be more efficient, with a resultant lowering of the resting and submaximal exercise heart rate and blood pressure. This, in turn, increases exercise time and intensity tolerance. Blood volume, both in terms of plasma and hemoglobin, increases oxygen-carrying capacity. Lactic acid metabolism also improves, allowing the aerobic system to break it down more effectively for usable energy, and muscle glycogen storage increases. Vasculature also increases so blood perfusion of muscles improves. Other positive adaptations include increased bone mineral density, improvements in body composition, and neural adaptations.

Cardiovascular Equipment

Strength coaches can make use of a variety of cardiovascular machines such as treadmills, bicycles, rowing machines, stair steppers, elliptical trainers, arm ergometers, and Arc trainers. The choice of the equipment may depend on the athlete's sport, training goals, availability, preference, injury, and workout plan. Coaches should teach athletes how to use the console, properly program the machine with the various inputs, and the proper form for each piece of equipment. For example, it is a common mistake to set an improper seat height on spin bikes and stationary bikes, often resulting in a seat that is too low, a knee that is too flexed, and a less-efficient stride. Athletes should set the seat height so that they fully extend their knee and straighten the leg downward. From there, they should lower the seat so that there is about 10 degrees of knee flexion at the lowest point in the cycle rotation.

Machine Programming and Setup

Many cardiovascular machines have programmable workouts such as intervals, hills, and tempo sessions. They may even record heart rate to gauge intensity, or athletes may select manual or free mode. These programming options are chosen at the beginning of the workout and inputted into the console along with age, weight, and workout duration. Resistance, speed, and incline can be changed during the workout. There is often a safety button or clip, which should be engaged for safety. Spin bikes use a dial that can change the relative resistance on the flywheel.

Preparatory Body and Limb Position

Athletes should use normal, healthy posture whether seated or standing and refrain from leaning on handrails. The spine should be in optimal alignment, with shoulders back and chest open. Athletes should avoid reading or watching video if it compromises form or causes slouching. On elliptical machines that include arm pedals, the elbows should be flexed to roughly 90 degrees, hands should have a neutral grip, and shoulders should remain relaxed. A recumbent bike can be used when the torso needs significant support; for example, in cases of upper extremity injury or rib fracture. However, in terms of cardiovascular benefit, this machine typically falls significantly short of other modes. On all cycle types, athletes should keep their torso upright and refrain from oscillating from side to side with each alternating pedal stroke. Pedal rate should typically mimic that of running at about 90 revolutions per minute, unless the athlete is specifically working on turnover, in which case the resistance can be lowered and over-speed training can occur. Some bikes display metabolic equivalents (METs), which serve as an indication of energy expenditure over that at rest and can be used as a gauge of intensity. Resistance coupled with speed factor into bicycling METs, while body weight, incline, and speed (pace) influence metabolic equivalents during treadmill running. An arm ergometer can be a good choice in cases of severe lower extremity injury or disability, or for athletes who need to work on upper body strength and muscular endurance, such as gymnasts and swimmers. This machine involves sitting upright in the provided chair and pedaling with the arms, much in the same way a normal bicycle functions with the legs.

Execution of Technique
Proper technique on cardiovascular equipment should parallel the technique used for the same activity outdoors. For example, runners on a treadmill should use arms flexed comfortably at the side, refraining from swinging them excessively across the midline. The feet should land at midfoot and not plod heavily on the heels; the body should be upright with good posture without a slouch, with a slight forward lean if the treadmill is set on an incline. Athletes should use steady, constant breathing, avoiding gasping and hyperventilating. If a workout is too intense and oxygen demand cannot keep up with oxygen supply, intensity may need to be reduced, unless it is designed to be an anaerobic interval. Particularly when athletes are injured and using cardiovascular equipment to cross train, they can use visualization techniques during the activity to practice mental imagery and focus.

Correction of Improper Technique
Coaches should ensure that athletes are using proper form and focusing on the workout at hand. There is a tendency for athletes to "zone out" on cardiovascular equipment in an attempt to distract themselves, so coaches should stress the importance of proper form, the goal of the workout, and the role of the exercise within the training program. Strength coaches should correct improper technique as early as possible in the learning process to prevent the development of bad habits and reduce risk of injury.

General 'Body-Only' Activities
"Body-Only" exercises such as running, swimming, walking, and dance are easy modalities for athletes to implement in their training programs when they are away from the gym and its various equipment. Most sports involve some amount of running as well, so this activity is particularly important for training. Swimming provides an excellent cross training activity because it improves cardiovascular and muscular fitness while reducing stress on joints and tissues in a non-weight-bearing environment. Strength coaches may supplement training with body-only activities, especially during the off-season or breaks from school when athletes might not have easy access to a training facility.

Execution of Technique
Running and walking technique are fairly innate and can be somewhat difficult to modify, especially in older athletes. However, strength coaches should evaluate running form for any obvious aberrations that might increase injury risk such as heel strike, over-striding, excessive or insufficient arm swing, or hunched posture. Cadence should be roughly 90 steps per minute per leg for most healthy athletes regardless of absolute speed. Swimming requires a great deal of technique, so strength coaches may need to defer to swimming coaches for proper instruction. Swimming economy and efficiency are greatly improved with proper form, breathing technique, arm pull, and kicking pattern. In the absence of solid technique, many highly trained athletes struggle significantly with endurance swimming, so individualized critique of form and drills might need to be implemented. It is optimal for athletes to learn to breathe on both sides during freestyle swimming.

Correction of Improper Technique
Video analysis of running form and swimming form might help in the coaching and correction of improper form. Specialized swimming coaches can be useful for giving pointers on improving technique. As with other aspects of training, strength coaches should correct improper technique as early as possible in the learning process to prevent the development of bad habits and to reduce risk of injury. Even advanced athletes may demonstrate poor technique when fatigued, distracted, or unmotivated, so observing and giving cues on preparatory and execution form technique needs to be a constant focus of strength coaches during workouts. For maximal effectiveness, feedback should be as specific and timely as possible, and should be visual, auditory, and kinesthetic, depending on each athlete's learning style.

Strength coaches may position athletes in front of the mirror so they can observe and self-correct deviations in form, sometimes concurrent with a proper form demonstration alongside the athlete for comparison. Coaches can also pair up athletes with differing skill levels to promote a learning/teaching mentorship. This can also help more experienced athletes develop leadership roles, while also finding a reason to focus on their own form, which may need some fine-tuning as the athlete becomes complacent with experience. Regardless of delivery method, all form correction feedback should be positive, supportive, and instructive to foster a warm learning environment and keep the athlete motivated and comfortable.

Anaerobic Conditioning Activities
There is a wide variety of anaerobic training techniques, often implementing intervals (periods of high-intensity activity interspersed with recovery rest periods): heavy battle ropes, jumping rope, climbing hills and stairs, line sprints or surges, and high-intensity conditioning drills such as jump squats, burpees, and high knees. Almost all sports have some degree of reliance on anaerobic energy systems, so this form of training needs to be prioritized in strength and conditioning programs.

Execution of Technique
Proper form is especially important during high-intensity activities when muscles, joints, tendons, and ligaments are under very high loads and speeds, subjecting them to increased force and demanding power. Strength coaches should instruct athletes to land all jumps with soft and slightly flexed knees, to pump arms powerfully and efficiently, and to breathe as much as possible. Even though these activities are not consuming a significant amount of oxygen due to their intensity and reliance on anaerobic metabolism, focusing on adequate breathing helps to maintain proper form and assists in a more rapid and comfortable recovery to quickly oxygenate the muscles and metabolic byproducts of anaerobic metabolism. When running stairs or uphill sprints, athletes should lift knees as high as possible. They should maintain a slight forward lean from the ankles and not the waist, and use aggressive, powerful arm swings. When descending, steps should be light and quick. Slight knee flexion will help protect knee cartilage and ligaments. Some athletes might choose to walk down hills backwards or otherwise mix up the downhill routine.

Heavy battle ropes are a great training tool for a total body workout, upper body power, endurance, and anaerobic bouts. There is a wide variety of exercises and patterns that can be implemented. A proper athletic stance should be encouraged, with the good squatting form of knees flexed, hips staying back behind the ankles, erect spine, good posture, chest up and out, and eyes forward. Most anaerobic activities are short enough in duration that athletes should be able to maintain mental focus on sustaining intensity and using good form throughout the duration. Coaches should provide adequate recovery between bouts of heavy exertion to ensure that athletes are able to truly maximize their efforts on each attempt.

Correction of Improper Technique
Coaches should monitor athletes for improper form and correct it as soon as possible, even stopping an interval early rather than letting the athlete continue with possibly injury-inducing form mistakes. Particularly with inadequate rest or increasing fatigue, form is likely to break down, even in athletes who are skilled. In these cases, workouts might need to be shortened, or rest intervals might need to be prolonged to keep the athlete performing with proper form to reap the maximum benefits of the programmed workout.

Flexibility Exercise Technique

Flexibility exercises can help improve range of motion, prevent injury, and prevent muscle, ligamentous, and tendon tightening. They also have a positive impact on elements of the nervous system, such as the Golgi tendon organs and mechanoreceptors, and they prepare the body to recruit the necessary motor units for optimal athletic performance. Athletes should receive coaching on proper and improper stretching techniques and instruction to hold a position in a comfortable and moderate stretch without causing pain.

Static Stretching Exercises
Static stretches should follow the completion of the workout, especially for excessively stiff athletes or those with previous injuries. Static stretching exercises can improve the muscle tension and joint relationship over time. Static stretches done prior to exercise can reduce explosive power and increase joint laxity when stiffness is required for energy conservation, placing an athlete at greater risk of injury.

Preparatory Body and Limb Position
Static stretching should take place after the workout while the muscles are warm. There is a variety of static stretches, most targeting the major muscles of the body. Some can be completed standing, such as the standing quadriceps stretch with the foot coming up behind the buttocks, stretches for the shoulders and chest, and standing hamstring and calf stretches. Seated stretches are mostly for the hips, glutes, and hamstrings. Supine stretches can be for the quadriceps, low back, and abdominals. During all static stretches, the athlete should be instructed to maintain good posture and joint alignment to keep joints within their normal range of motion (ROM) without hyperextension, and to keep them within their typical planes of motion (i.e., sagittal plane for flexion) without undue twisting and contorting.

Execution of Technique
Stretches are typically held at the end range of motion for 30 seconds, followed by a brief rest, then repeated for 2-3 total sets. The body should be held as still as possible, refraining from any bouncing or excessive reaching and relaxing. The joints should always be in safe, anatomically-normal positions (i.e., without hyperextending or twisting out of typical planes of motion). For example, the traditional hurdler's stretch, with one leg extended in front of the body and the other knee bent with the foot back behind the buttocks, twists the knee and can damage ligaments and is therefore contraindicated. Breathing should be smooth and steady, and athletes should focus on the tension in the muscles and imagine elongating and releasing the tension.

Correction of Improper Technique
To correct improper technique and prevent injuries, strength coaches should watch for ballistic, bouncing movements, joints that are twisted or hyperextended, and athletes who are grimacing or otherwise showing signs of excessive stretching.

Proprioceptive Neuromuscular Facilitation (PNF) Stretching Exercises
Proprioceptive Neuromuscular Facilitation (PNF) is a technique that uses the neuromuscular responses to specific feedback from isometric and concentric contractions performed both actively and passively. These actions and responses result in changes in the muscle/joint tension relationships and enable greater ROM to be achieved. In this way, PNF uses neurological phenomena to facilitate muscular inhibition in a specific protocol designed to improve flexibility and decrease discomfort from stretching. PNF relies on autogenic inhibition whereby inhibitory signals from the Golgi tendon organs override the excitatory impulses from the muscle spindles, resulting in gradual relaxation of the muscle. PNF is typically completed with a partner.

Preparatory Body and Limb Position
PNF stretching can be used for a variety of muscle groups such as the hamstrings, quadriceps, chest, and shoulder muscles. Positions vary depending on the muscle stretched. For example, hamstrings are done with the athlete in the supine position.

Body Mechanics to Perform PNF Stretching on an Athlete
The partner or coach must not only apply appropriate resistance for the stretching athlete, but also must be in the correct position, typically at the end range of the desired movement with the facilitator's shoulders and hips facing the direction of movement. How the facilitator moves directly influences how the athlete moves. The desired movement should bisect the facilitator's midline and center of gravity. The strength coach's body should be positioned in such a way that the resistance applied to the athlete should come from the trunk and hips, not the extremities.

Execution of Technique
There are three forms of PNF stretching: hold-relax, contract-relax, and hold-relax with agonist contraction, which all begin with 10-seconds of passive pre-stretch held at the point of mild discomfort. In the hold-relax, after the pre-stretch, the partner applies a flexion force while the athlete holds and tries to resist the force, creating an isometric contraction for 6 seconds. The athlete then relaxes back into a passive stretch lasting 30 seconds, which is now a deeper stretch than the initial pre-stretch due to autogenic inhibition. Using the hamstrings as an example, in the contract-relax method after the pre-stretch, the athlete extends the hip while the partner resists this extension so that a concentric contraction occurs throughout the full ROM. After this, the athlete relaxes back into a passive hip flexion stretch of 30 seconds in duration, again deeper than initially performed due to autogenic inhibition (activation of the hamstrings, in this case). The hold-relax with the agonist contraction uses the idea of reciprocal inhibition, whereby the contraction of the agonist muscle causes relaxation of the antagonist so that after the regular hold-relax protocol, the second passive stretch is replaced with an active stretch to further increase the stretch.

Here are some examples:

Hold-Relax PNF Technique for Hamstrings

1. Passive stretch

2. Contract against resistance

3. Relax ... Passive stretch

Correction of Improper Technique
It is important that both the athlete and the partner or strength coach are in the proper positions and using correct techniques to effectively and safely use PNF. Coaches can get injured as well, if they attempt to provide resistance from their extremities rather than through the hips and trunk. They also must be sure to keep the hips and shoulders squarely facing the direction of movement to not induce any twisting of the spine. Athletes should be instructed to breathe and only push stretches to the point of mild discomfort to prevent overstretching. Because PNF relies on overriding neural regulation of the stretch reflex, it is important to exactly follow the protocols to protect the tendons and muscles. Strength coaches should pay extra attention to athletes nursing injuries or those with hypermobile joints.

Dynamic Stretching Exercises
Dynamic stretching or mobility drills emphasize the required movements of the planned activity – rather than individual muscles – by actively moving the joint through the ROM encountered in a sport prior to the sport. Dynamic stretching occurs before the activity as part of the warm-up routine to increase heart rate, temperature, and blood flow, as well as CNS (central nervous system) and PNS (peripheral nervous system) activity to prepare the body. It promotes dynamic flexibility and mimics the movement patterns

and ROM needed in sports activities without ballistic movements. It is less effective than static PNF stretching on increasing static ROM.

Preparatory Body and Limb Position
A neutral erect spine and athletic posture should be maintained in dynamic stretching or mobility drills. Drills such as walking lunges and hip mobility drills should use proper squatting form.

Execution of Technique
Athletes typically complete 5-10 repetitions of each movement, either in place or over a given distance with a progressive increase in the ROM and/or speed on each repetition or set. The movement mechanics of the sport should be reinforced in the mobility drill, along with the predominant joint positions, such as ankle dorsiflexion on a high knee drill for sprinters.

Correction of Improper Technique
Coaches should ensure that athletes move deliberately and progressively through the ROM, but in a controlled fashion that does not include bouncing. The focus should always be on proper technique and form while warming up the body and perfecting sport-specific movements.

Spotting Procedures and Techniques

Spotting procedures help athletes complete exercises safely and efficiently. Not only do coaches need to know how to execute correct spotting techniques, but they must be able to demonstrate and teach the techniques to athletes so that they can spot one another during partner activities. Spotting also helps monitor an athlete's lifting form and movement execution, allowing the spotter to give verbal cues and help correct any errors in execution. It also allows for motivation, instruction, encouragement, feedback, and certain exercise modifications that would otherwise not only be dangerous, but physically impossible, without spotters. An example is negative resistance training, wherein athletes can handle greater weight on the eccentric or lowering portion, but need spotters to help raise the weight in the concentric phase. Spotters should be prepared to offer as much help as needed. Clear communication between the lifter and spotter is required for safety, and the pair should discuss the lift before it occurs. The spotter should ensure that the weights are evenly spaced and equally loaded on the bar and that the collars are properly used.

<u>Number of Spotters Needed for Given Situations and Exercises</u>
The required number of spotters is determined by the load being lifted, the experience and skill of the athlete and spotters, and the physical strength of the spotters. The spotters must be strong enough to handle the load that the athlete is lifting with little notice and sometimes in less than ideal angles and positions. Therefore, it is crucial that spotters are honest with themselves and lifters about their abilities. It is better to err on the side of caution and use multiple spotters when necessary, as long as they can be accommodated spatially around the lift without being overly cumbersome. With the exception of power exercises, free weight exercises should use a minimum of one or two spotters when an athlete moves the bar over the head or face, or has it on the front of the shoulders or positioned on the back during the execution. During power exercises, athlete should be instructed to push the bar away or drop it when the bar is in front, and release it or jump forward when the bar is missed behind the head. A spotter should not be used. Two spotters are sometimes needed with heavy lifts, especially bar lifts, where one spotter should be at each end of the bar.

<u>Spotter Location</u>
The location of the spotter or spotters depends on the lift being attempted. For exercises with heavy weights on a bar such as a front squat, often two spotters are needed at each end of the bar to help

balance the weight with the athlete and lift from either side, should an issue occur. For standing exercises such as squats and deadlifts, spotters should stand behind the lifter while the bar is still on the rack and as the lifter gets into position. They should then move as close as possible toward the lifter without touching him or her, as the lifter steps away from the rack with the bar. The spotter's hands should be in the ready position near the bar while the lifter raises and lowers the weight. Once the set is complete or when failure is indicated by the lifter, the spotter should assist the lifter in returning the bar to the rack by holding onto the bar and guiding it back to the racked position. During exercises such as a dumbbell bench press, spotters should keep their hands near the lifter's forearms, close to the wrists. For a seated overhead triceps extension with a barbell, spotters should straddle the flat bench.

Body and Limb Placement Required When Spotting the Lifter
Once the spotter and the lifter are in the correct positions, the spotter needs to pay attention to their body and limb placement for their own safety during the lift as well as that of the athlete. When spotting over-the-face barbell exercises, the spotter should grasp the bar with an alternated grip, usually narrower than that of the athlete's grip. The spotter also should use a solid, wide base of support and a neutral spine position. Spotters should use an athletic stance, with feet slightly wider than hip-width apart, knees flexed, arms and hands up and in a ready position that is close to the bar and athlete without touching them. Bodyweight should be equally and soundly distributed on both feet, which should be firmly planted on the ground. Spotters must follow the movement of the athlete and the bar with their eyes as well as their hands, and remain intensely focused on the task at hand until the bar is re-racked. Spotters and lifters should communicate throughout the lift if anything changes, but it is the spotter's job to verbally motivate and check in with the lifter, since the athlete is likely less physically and mentally able to talk during maximal exertion.

Practice Questions

1. Benefits of resistance machines include all BUT which of the following?
    a. They can be used easily without a spotter
    b. They can be particularly helpful for newer athletes to learn proper form and control the motion within the desired plane of movement
    c. They can improve sports-specific movements and strength, incorporating core stability
    d. Athletes can often lift higher maximal weights and isolate specific muscles, improving absolute strength

2. When using starting blocks for sprinting, which of the following best describes optimal hand position?
    a. Hands should be slightly less than shoulder-width apart with the fingers held together and thumbs under the shoulders.
    b. Hands should be slightly wider than shoulder-width apart with the fingers held together and thumbs under the shoulders.
    c. Hands should be slightly less than shoulder-width apart with the fingers spread apart and thumbs under the armpits.
    d. Hands should be slightly wider than shoulder-width apart with the fingers spread apart and thumbs under the armpits.

3. Box jumps, depth jumps, and medicine ball throws are examples of what type of training?
    a. Plyometrics
    b. Agility exercises
    c. Non-traditional modalities
    d. Speed training

4. During agility exercises, weight should be concentrated on what part of the foot?
    a. Forefoot
    b. Midfoot
    c. Hind foot
    d. Heel

5. Incorporating yoga training into an athlete's regimen can be beneficial in all BUT which of the following ways?
    a. It improves core strength
    b. It improves flexibility
    c. It improves mental focus and relaxation
    d. It improves absolute strength

6. Free weights have all of the following benefits over resistance machines EXCEPT which of the following?
    a. They should be completed with a spotter.
    b. They can improve core stability.
    c. They can provide a more sports-specific strength training method.
    d. Each exercise can be performed in a variety of ways, rather than strictly dictated in one certain way.

7. What is the most challenging part of a strength exercise called?
   a. Eccentric phase
   b. Concentric phase
   c. Sticking point
   d. Maximal point

8. For most strength exercises, which of the following breathing patterns is optimal?
   a. Inhale through the mouth during the concentric phase and exhale through the nose during the eccentric phase
   b. Exhale through the mouth during the concentric phase and inhale through the nose during the eccentric phase
   c. Inhale through the nose during the concentric phase and exhale through the mouth during the eccentric phase
   d. Exhale through the nose in the concentric phase and inhale through the mouth during the eccentric phase

9. Mirrors and video analysis can be helpful in which of the following ways?
   a. Correcting improper form
   b. Allowing a strength coach to focus less on monitoring athletes
   c. Correcting improper technique
   d. Providing visual feedback regarding form and technique

10. Which of the following is NOT an adaptation to chronic cardiovascular conditioning?
    a. Increased heart chamber size
    b. Increased stroke volume
    c. Increased cardiac output
    d. Increased submaximal heart rate

11. Depth achieved during a squat is often limited by which of the following?
    a. Knee injuries
    b. Hamstring tightness
    c. Achilles tendon tightness
    d. Gastrocnemius (calf) weakness

12. When using free weights, how many points of contact should be made for supine and seated exercises?
    a. 2
    b. 3
    c. 4
    d. 5

13. Which direction should the palms face when using a supinated grip?
    a. Upward toward the face
    b. Downwards toward the feet
    c. Inward toward the hips
    d. Out laterally away from the body

14. Which athlete would benefit most from agility work on most days of the week?
    a. A soccer midfielder
    b. A baseball pitcher
    c. A shot putter
    d. A swimmer

15. Which athlete would benefit most from plyometrics at least three days per week?
    a. A cross country runner
    b. A hockey player
    c. A figure skater
    d. A swimmer

16. What is the name for the grip pattern where palms face the floor and the knuckles face the ceiling?
    a. Pronated grip
    b. Supinated grip
    c. Hook grip
    d. False grip

17. Golgi tendon organs are stimulated in PNF stretching and cause relaxation of which of the following?
    a. The antagonist muscle by its own contraction
    b. The stretched muscle by its own contraction
    c. The antagonist muscle by contracting the stretched muscle
    d. The stretched muscle by contracting the antagonist muscle

18. Activation of muscle spindles is decreased in which of the following stretching methods?
    a. Dynamic
    b. Passive
    c. Static
    d. PNF

19. In order of decreasing percentage of total training volume, for a distance runner's program, which of the following would you suggest for the given activities?
    a. Cardiovascular/metabolic conditioning, muscular endurance, agility training, plyometrics
    b. Cardiovascular/metabolic conditioning, muscular endurance, plyometrics, agility training
    c. Cardiovascular/metabolic conditioning, agility training, muscular endurance, plyometrics
    d. Cardiovascular/metabolic conditioning, plyometrics, muscular endurance, agility training

20. In order of decreasing frequency for a tennis player's training program, which of the following would you suggest for the given activities?
    a. Speed training, cardiovascular conditioning, plyometrics, agility training
    b. Cardiovascular conditioning, speed training, agility training, plyometrics
    c. Cardiovascular conditioning, agility training, speed training, plyometrics
    d. Agility training, speed training, plyometrics, cardiovascular conditioning

21. All BUT which of the following are forms of PNF technique?
    a. Contract-relax
    b. Contract-relax with agonist contraction
    c. Hold-relax with agonist contraction
    d. Hold-relax

22. Which of the following is the correct protocol for the hold-relax PNF technique?
    a. 10-second passive pre-stretch, isometric contraction for 6 seconds, passive stretch for 30 seconds
    b. 10-second passive pre-stretch, isometric contraction for 6 seconds, passive stretch for 10 seconds
    c. 6-second passive pre-stretch, isometric contraction for 10 seconds, passive stretch for 30 seconds
    d. 6-second passive pre-stretch, isometric contraction for 10 seconds, passive stretch for 10 seconds

23. Benefits of static stretching include all EXCEPT which of the following?
    a. It improves muscle-joint tension relationship
    b. It can warm up muscles prior to workout
    c. It can increase joint laxity
    d. It can reduce risk of injury

24. With which of the following athletes should you use extra precaution when programming plyometric exercises?
    a. A distance runner
    b. A 250-pound lineman
    c. A female athlete
    d. A figure skater

25. Which of the following anatomic structures detects rapid movement and initiates the stretch reflex?
    a. Extrafusal muscle fibers
    b. Mechanoreceptors
    c. Golgi tendon organs
    d. Muscle spindles

26. Static stretches should be held for about how many seconds and for how many sets?
    a. 30, 2-3
    b. 30, 3-5
    c. 10, 2-3
    d. 10, 3-5

27. Tire flipping, kettlebells, sandbags, and battle ropes are implements best reserved for which of the following?
    a. Highly trained athletes
    b. Younger athletes
    c. Athletes rehabbing injuries
    d. Newer athletes

28. Which type of stretching should be done prior to workouts and which type of stretching should follow the workout?
    a. Static, dynamic
    b. Dynamic, static
    c. Flexibility, dynamic
    d. Dynamic, flexibility

29. Which of the following factors is most influential in improving sprinting speed?
    a. Leg length
    b. Stride length
    c. Stride rate
    d. Impulse time

30. An athlete has medial tibial stress syndrome, which of the following cardiovascular equipment is NOT a wise choice?
    a. Arm ergometer
    b. Elliptical
    c. Spin bike
    d. Treadmill

31. Spotters should be used for all EXCEPT which of the following exercises?
    a. Dumbbell chest press
    b. Incline barbell bench press
    c. Front squat
    d. Power jerk

32. Benefits of the Valsalva maneuver include all EXCEPT which of the following?
    a. Increases blood pressure
    b. Increases torso rigidity
    c. Decreases compressive forces on the intervertebral disks
    d. Supports the normal lordotic lumbar spine

33. During a heavy front-loaded squat, there should be how many spotter(s) who should be positioned in what location?
    a. 1, in the middle of the bar in front of the lifter
    b. 1, in the middle of the bar behind the lifter
    c. 2, on either end of the bar
    d. 2, one in front of and one behind the lifter

34. The number of required spotters is dependent on all EXCEPT which of the following?
    a. The load being lifted
    b. The number of strength coaches available
    c. The experience and skill of the athlete and spotters
    d. The physical strength of the spotters

35. When spotting over-the-face barbell exercises, the spotter should use what type of grip on the bar?
    a. Hook grip
    b. Pronated grip
    c. Alternated grip
    d. Supinated grip

36. Correct spotting position includes all BUT which of the following?
    a. Knees locked
    b. Feet flat on the floor
    c. Hands up in ready position
    d. Erect, neutral spine

37. Negative resistance training is best described as which of the following?
    a. Reducing training volume prior to competition to taper and improve performance
    b. A detraining effect that occurs when athletes fail to train with high enough frequency
    c. Lifting heavier weights on the lowering, eccentric portion and getting assistance during the lifting, concentric phase
    d. Lifting heavier weights on the lifting, concentric portion and getting assistance during the lowering, eccentric phase

38. Benefits of bodyweight exercises include all BUT which of the following?
    a. They increase relative strength
    b. They increase absolute strength
    c. They can be performed on the field or away from the gym
    d. Athletes can often complete many repetitions, improving muscular endurance

Answer Explanations

1. C: Because resistance machines are often used in the seated position and they only allow movement in one given plane, the core does not need to work to stabilize the body and they do not improve sports-specific skills as well as free weights. Benefits of resistance machines include the fact that they can be used more easily without a spotter, they can be particularly helpful for newer athletes to learn proper form and control the motion within the desired plane of movement, and due to the support they provide, athletes can often lift higher maximal weights and isolate specific muscles, improving absolute strength.

2. B: When using starting blocks for sprinting, the athlete should place his or her hands just behind the starting line slightly wider than shoulder-width apart with the fingers held together. The thumb should bridge out to the side and should by directly under the shoulders, ready to support bodyweight.

3. A: Box jumps, depth jumps, and medicine ball throws are examples of plyometrics. Agility exercises include things such as ladder drills and cones; non-traditional modalities might include kettlebells, heavy ropes, and tires; and speed training involves sprint training and foot drills.

4. A: During agility exercises, weight should be concentrated on the forefoot to allow for quick movements and changes in direction.

5. D: Incorporating yoga training into an athlete regimen can be beneficial for improving core strength, flexibility, and mental focus and relaxation. Because it involves bodyweight only, it improves relative strength but not absolute strength.

6. A: Exercises with free weights should use a minimum of one or two spotters when an athlete moves the bar over the head or face, has it on the front of the shoulders, or has it on the back during the execution. Resistance machines frequently do not need a spotter because they have safety features designed into them, but for certain maximal lifts, a spotter is recommended. Free weight training can improve core stability and can provide a more sports-specific strength training method. Each exercise can be performed in a variety of ways, rather than strictly dictated in one specific way.

7. C: The most challenging part of a strength exercise is called the sticking point. In a bench press, this is where the direction of the bar changes from coming down toward the chest to then being pushed back away.

8. B: For most strength exercises, the athlete should exhale through the mouth during the concentric phase through the sticking point and then inhale through the nose during the eccentric phase. Breathing should be slow and controlled.

9. D: Mirrors and video analysis can be used to provide visual feedback regarding form and technique to guide corrections. They do not correct form or technique in and of themselves, but are useful tools to help identify such issues and begin the process of correcting improper technique. For safety and to reduce liability, strength coaches should always focus on monitoring athletes.

10. D: Increased submaximal heart rate is not a chronic adaptation to cardiovascular exercise. In fact, heart rate decreases at a given submaximal workload due to improvements in cardiorespiratory economy. Heart chamber size increases, as does preload (the amount of blood that fills a chamber before it contracts to eject it), resulting in a higher stroke volume per heartbeat. This means that more blood, oxygen, and nutrients get moved per pump of the heart. Blood volume and hemoglobin content of the blood also increase.

11. C: Depth of squats is often limited by Achilles tendon tightness. For athletes who are limited in squat depth due to tight Achilles tendons, elevating the heels on a weight plate or other incline will help achieve a deeper squat, despite limited range of motion in the ankles.

12. D: Exercises in the seated and supine positions require five points of contact for optimal body support: the head is firmly situated on the bench or back pad, the shoulders and upper back are evenly placed firmly on the bench or back pad, the buttocks are positioned evenly on the bench or seat, and the right and left foot are both placed flat on the floor.

13. A: In a supinated grip, palms face upward toward the face and knuckles face the floor. In a pronated grip, knuckles are up and palms face the floor.

14. A: Soccer requires a great deal of agility, so these athletes benefit from agility work on most days in each training cycle. Because agility technique takes a high degree of focus and cognition, it is best to complete it in high-frequency, short-duration sessions in a training program. This is usually accomplished by short agility drill sessions most days of the week.

15. B: Hockey players need to have significant explosive power, strength, and speed, so they benefit greatly from plyometrics, which develop explosive power. Three days per week is about the maximum frequency that is recommended for plyometrics, given their intensity and the demand they place on the anatomic structures of the body and physiologic systems. Beyond this, there is increased risk of injury, even in experienced athletes. Most athletes can benefit from some plyometric training, but such a frequency is not needed for the endurance athletes listed.

16. A: The grip pattern where palms face the floor and the knuckles face the ceiling is called a pronated grip.

17. B: Golgi tendon organs are stimulated in PNF stretching and cause relaxation of the stretched muscle by its own contraction.

18. D: Activation of muscle spindles is decreased in PNF stretching, which capitalizes autogenic inhibition to send inhibitory signals from the Golgi tendon organs to the brain. These inhibitory signals override the excitatory impulses from the muscle spindles, which causes the muscle to gradually relax. Normally, stimulation of muscle spindles induces a contraction of the stretched muscle.

19. B: In order of decreasing percentage of total training volume, for a distance runner's program, cardiovascular/metabolic conditioning should be prioritized because this forms the foundation of the runner's fitness, followed by muscular endurance, which is also needed for endurance running. Plyometrics will help build some power, strength, and speed, and may help strengthen the anatomy to prevent injuries. Agility is least necessary as a focus for endurance runners, since they are mostly trying not to change speed or direction, and especially because the question is asking about percentage of volume and not frequency.

20. C: This question was tricky because it is asking about the frequency of various components of training, so you needed to not only focus on the specifics of tennis, but keep in mind general guidelines for frequency of types of training in a program. Tennis requires strong cardiovascular fitness, so this should form the foundation of the training program and not only comprise the most volume, but also frequency, since some amount of aerobic conditioning should occur on essentially all training days in a program. Speed and agility are incredibly important for successful tennis playing as well; it is here that planning safe programming in terms of frequency comes into play. Speed training likely should take on a larger percentage of training volume (a greater number of total minutes dedicated to speed training during the week compared to agility), but speed training should be limited to just a few days per week to allow the body to fully recover from the demands and damage it causes. Agility is best completed in short, frequent bouts due to its high cognitive demand. Therefore, agility should occur more frequently than speed training. Plyometrics develop explosive power, which is important for tennis players, but should be limited to two days per week to prevent injury from overtraining and overstressing the anatomy.

21. B: There are three forms of PNF stretching: hold-relax, contract-relax, and hold-relax with agonist contraction, which all begin with 10-seconds of passive pre-stretch held at the point of mild discomfort. In the hold-relax, after the pre-stretch, the partner applies a flexion force while the athlete holds and tries to resist the force, creating an isometric contraction for 6 seconds, then the athlete relaxes back into a passive stretch lasting 30 seconds, which is now a deeper stretch than the initial pre-stretch due to autogenic inhibition. The hold-relax with the agonist contraction uses the idea of reciprocal inhibition whereby the contraction of the agonist muscle causes relaxation of the antagonist. Therefore, after the regular hold-relax protocol, the second passive stretch is replaced with an active stretch to further increase stretch.

22. A: The hold-relax PNF protocol begins with a 10-second passive pre-stretch held at the point of mild discomfort. Then the partner applies a flexion force while the athlete holds and tries to resist the force, creating an isometric contraction for 6 seconds. After this, the athlete relaxes back into a passive stretch lasting 30 seconds. This is now a deeper stretch than the initial pre-stretch due to autogenic inhibition.

23. B: Static stretches should follow the workout, especially for excessively stiff athletes or those with past injuries. It can improve the muscle tension and joint relationship over time. Static stretches performed prior to exercise can reduce explosive power and increase joint laxity when stiffness is required for energy conservation, placing an athlete at greater risk of injury.

24. B: While care and caution should be employed for all athletes doing plyometrics, the football player poses the greatest risk of injury due to his weight. Because of the demand on the body, proper technique is imperative to avoid injury. Heavier athletes (over 220 pounds) should also be monitored for any joint tenderness because the forces on their joints coupled with the weight of the body can place excessive stress on the tissues. Special care must be considered for previously injured athletes, senior athletes, prepubescents, and those with balance issues. Proper footwear and soft, rubberized flooring or grass should be used to reduce landing forces.

25. D: Muscle spindles detect rapid movement and initiate the stretch reflex. Golgi tendon organs are a type of mechanoreceptors that control the flexibility and extensibility of the muscles and joints when they are stretched or during reactive forces or muscular contractions. Extrafusal fibers are the main skeletal muscle fibers in a muscle.

26. A: Static stretches should be held for about 30 seconds and in 2-3 sets for maximal efficacy. They should follow a workout for athletes with chronic tightness, and not precede it.

27. A: Tire flipping, kettlebells, sandbags, and battle ropes are implements best reserved for highly trained athletes. Such implements are creative ways to add variety to workouts while accomplishing similar physiologic goals. Coaches must still be aware of when and how to properly use this equipment and be sure to educate and supervise athletes in its use. Much of the non-traditional equipment is best reserved for advanced athletes who have the basic foundations of movement, such as a well-mastered squat and deadlift, because programs with non-traditional equipment tend to use heavier implements in power movements, which can induce injury if not carried out safely.

28. B: Dynamic stretching should be done prior to workouts and static stretching should follow the workout. Dynamic stretching occurs before the activity as part of the warm-up routine to increase heart rate, temperature, and blood flow, as well as CNS and PNS activity to prepare the body. Static stretches should follow the workout, especially for excessively stiff athletes or those with past injuries. Static stretching can improve the muscle tension and joint relationship over time. Static stretches performed prior to exercise can reduce explosive power and increase joint laxity, placing an athlete at greater risk of injury.

29. C: Speed is influenced by stride rate and stride length, so athletes should focus on quick turnover and powerful steps. Of these factors, stride rate has a greater impact on speed and should be the focus when designing programming for improving sprinting speed. Leg length cannot be readily modified, especially after growth has ceased.

30. D: Medial tibial stress syndrome, or shin splints, is an overuse injury made worse by pounding or impact, so treadmill running should be avoided. Non-weight bearing cardiovascular equipment such as an arm ergometer or bike is ideal. The elliptical can be a workable option as long as it does not cause pain. It is weight-bearing, but non-impact.

31. D: Spotters are not used in power exercises such as the power jerk. With the exception of power exercises, free weight exercises should use a minimum of one or two spotters when an athlete moves the bar over the head or face, has it on the front of the shoulders, or on the back during the execution. During power exercises, athlete should be instructed to push the bar away or drop it when the bar is in front, and release it or jump forward when the bar is missed behind the head; a spotter should not be used.

32. A: The Valsalva maneuver can be used in certain core exercises with care as a way to increase torso rigidity to aid in support of the vertebral column, which lessens compressive forces on the intervertebral discs and supports the normal and neutral lordotic lumbar spine. Blood pressure can increase with the Valsalva maneuver, but this is not a benefit, and in fact, can cause undesirable dizziness and disorientation.

33. C: During a heavy front-loaded squat, there should be 2 spotters – one positioned on either end of the bar – to help balance it and to remain in constant communication with each other and the lifter.

34. B: The required number of spotters is determined by the load being lifted, the experience and skill of the athlete and spotters, and the physical strength of the spotters. The spotters must be strong enough to handle the load that the athlete is lifting with little notice and sometimes in less than ideal angles and positions, so it is crucial that spotters are honest with themselves and the lifter about their abilities. It is safer to err on the side of caution and use multiple spotters when necessary, as long as they can be accommodated spatially around the lift without being overly cumbersome.

35. C: When spotting over-the-face barbell exercises, the spotter should use the alternated grip pattern, usually narrower than the athlete's grip. In this position, one hand is supinated and one is pronated.

36. A: Spotters should use a solid, wide base of support and a neutral spine position. Spotters should use an athletic stance, with feet slightly wider than hip width apart, knees flexed, arms and hands up and in the ready position and as close to the bar and athlete without touching them as possible. Bodyweight should be equally and soundly distributed on both feet, which should be firmly planted on the ground. Knees should not be locked but should maintain a degree of flexion, ready to support the weight and go into a squat if necessary to accept the weight of the bar. Locking the knees can be dangerous, since it places excessive stress on the knee ligaments and cartilage as well as the lower leg muscles and bones and the low back.

37. C: Negative resistance training is best described as lifting heavier weights on the lowering, eccentric portion and getting assistance from spotters during the lifting, concentric phase. It is a specific resistance training protocol based on the concept that most athletes can handle heavier loads on the eccentric portions of exercises, but are not able to lift the load concentrically, so they need assistance. However, if they are only to use the load they can handle concentrically, they are never fully challenging the stronger eccentrically working muscles, so negative resistance training addresses this discrepancy. It is an advanced lifting technique.

38. B: Bodyweight training such as pull-ups, push-ups, chin-ups, squat thrusts, lunges, yoga, jumping jacks, and planks provide resistance in the form of bodyweight, so it improves relative strength and core strength, is low-cost, and improves body control. Because there are not external weights used, it does not improve absolute strength.

Program Design

Program Design

The first step in designing an appropriate program for an athlete is to create a needs analysis. The needs analysis helps the strength and conditioning professional to compare the requirements of the athlete's sport to the athlete's current fitness level. An athlete's ability to complete certain movement patterns will help identify any problems with body mechanics and specific muscle groups. Physiological tests will help the coach determine the demands that the athlete's sport places on the body, which can form the basis of a conditioning and resistance-training program. The athlete's history of injuries will also help the coach anticipate potential problems the athlete may have with certain muscle movements or exercise intensities.

Resistance Training

Free Weights
The source of resistance for free weights is gravity. Free-weight exercises are often performed in a standing position, which places more stress on the body's muscles and bones than weight-stack machines. Free weights require muscles to support and stabilize the body. Lifting free weights is a closer replication of the movements required in sports, because it involves the coordination of multiple muscle groups (as opposed to machines, which typically isolate single muscle groups).

Weight-Stack Machines
The source of resistance for weight-stack machines is gravity; however, these machines utilize cables, pulleys, cams, and gears that allow increased control over both the pattern and direction of resistance. Weight-stack machines are safer than free weights, in part because less skill and muscle coordination are needed for control, and the design of the machines provides resistance to body movements that are difficult to duplicate with free weights (e.g., hip adduction and abduction, or leg curl). Machines also can be readied more quickly than free weights because weight selection only requires inserting a pin into the weight stack.

Circuit Training
The use of circuit training during resistance-training sessions condenses the time needed to complete a specific amount of work. The athlete goes from one exercise to the next with limited rest between the movement sets. Circuit training can be used with any type of resistance exercise movement, but the most demanding movement sets (i.e., power movements) should be completed before less demanding movement sets (i.e., core and assistance movements). There are several benefits to using circuit training, including improved time efficiency, enhanced cardiorespiratory functioning, and increased muscle endurance. Circuit training increases metabolic costs and can be beneficial for athletes interested in reducing body fat.

Alternative Modes and Nontraditional Implement Training

Bodyweight-Training Methods
Bodyweight training is a basic resistance-training method that utilizes an individual's bodyweight as resistance. This training helps to develop core muscles and, as a result, may decrease injury risk. Benefits of bodyweight training include the following: bodyweight training is specific to the athlete's anthropometrics; it incorporates many closed chain exercises; it improves body control and relative strength while strengthening multiple muscle groups simultaneously; and it is a low-cost form of

training. The limitations of bodyweight training include the following: The load is limited by the athlete's weight; training does not substantially improve absolute strength; and changing movement patterns or repetitions is required to increase intensity. As the number of repetitions increases, the outcome focus of training will change from strength to strength endurance. Examples of bodyweight-training exercises include:

- Pull-ups
- Sit-ups
- Push-ups
- Squat thrusts
- Chin-ups
- Calisthenics
- Yoga
- Gymnastics

Core-Stability and Balance Training Methods
The scientific definition of the anatomical core is the axial skeleton (which includes the shoulder and pelvic girdles) and all of the soft tissues (i.e., muscles, articular cartilage, tendons, fascia, ligaments, and fibrocartilage).

Isolation Exercises
These exercises usually are dynamic or isometric muscle actions that isolate the specific core musculature. The upper and lower extremities do NOT contribute to the muscle actions. These exercises can improve spinal stability because there is increased muscle activation. Performance improvements may be seen in untrained athletes as well as athletes recovering from injury; however, research suggests that these exercises generally do not improve sport performance in other athlete populations. Research indicates that ground-based free-weight exercises (e.g., snatch, deadlift, squat, push-press, and trunk-rotation exercises) produce the same or greater levels of core-musculature activation. Examples of isolation exercises include:

- Side plank
- Prone plank

Instability Devices
Effects of Instability-Based Exercises
Instability-based exercises utilize unstable surfaces or devices to cause imbalances requiring increased stabilization functioning of the core musculature. While using these devices, the application of external forces to an individual's center of mass, called perturbations, can cause balance challenges that require core musculature to activate to make postural adjustments and maintain balance. Evidence indicates that core-musculature activation may increase with the use of instability devices. However, the agonist muscle has reduced force generation and a reduced rate of force development. Also, the overall power output and overall force-generating capacity may be 70% or less of that produced during exercise under stable conditions.

Effectiveness of Instability-Based Exercises Versus Ground-Based Exercises
The use of instability devices during static balance activities can help to improve balance and core stability before starting ground-based free-weight exercises done on stable surfaces. Ground-based free-weight exercises (e.g., Olympic lifts, squats) are a better exercise stimulus for developing core stability. These exercises have some inherent instability that facilitates the development of the links of

the kinetic chain, which helps improve sport performance to a greater extent than instability-based exercises.

Examples of instability devices include:

- Physio balls
- Hemispherical physio balls (BOSU)
- Inflatable disks
- Balance boards
- Wobble boards
- Foam tubes and platforms

Variable-Resistance Training Methods

Types of variable-resistance training methods include the following:

- Constant External Resistance: Constant external resistance involves free weights and traditional resistance exercises where the external load remains constant throughout the movement. This type of movement better replicates real activities and promotes more realistic movement patterns and skeletal muscle coordination.

- Accommodating Resistance: Also known as semi-isokinetic resistance applications, accommodating resistance controls the speed of movement (i.e., isokinetic resistance) throughout a range of motion (ROM). This type of training requires specific devices that generally have poor external validity and provide an inadequate training stimulus in comparison with constant external resistance exercises.

- Variable Resistance: Variable resistance training utilizes devices that apply varied resistance as the joint angle changes in an attempt to maximize forced application across the full ROM. Strength and conditioning facilities commonly combine chains or rubber bands with traditional free-weight resistance-training methods in order to alter the loading profile, thus allowing varied resistance across the ROM.

- Chain-Supplemented Exercises: Variable resistance can be applied by the addition of chains to resistance exercise activities (e.g., back squat or bench press). The size (e.g., diameter, length, density, or number of links) of the chain controls the amount of resistance it provides. The use of chains results in a linear increase in the applied resistance. Two ways to apply chains are to let them touch the floor from the fully extended position of the movement or to hang them from lighter chains so they only touch the floor when the lowest portion of the movement pattern (e.g., bottom of the squat) is reached.

  Note: Determining the Barbell Load to Use with Chains: First, an athlete must determine what the barbell load should be without chains. Second, the athlete should take the average of the chain resistance at the top and bottom of the movement. Third, the average chain resistance should be subtracted from the desired barbell load to determine the final barbell load. For example, an athlete who wants to train at a 5-RM (repetition-maximum) load on bench press must first determine the 5-RM load without the chains. If the 5-RM load without chains is 120 kg, then subtract the average chain resistance from this load. If the bottom position has a chain resistance of 0 kg and the top position has a chain resistance of 11.1 kg, the average chain resistance is 5.55 kg (11.1÷2). The athlete would need to subtract 5.55 kg from 120 kg to have appropriate barbell loading.

- Resistance-Band Exercises: There is some research supporting the efficacy of using resistance bands in combination with traditional resistance exercise. The strength and conditioning professional needs to be aware that the make-up of the resistance bands can affect their tension (resistance), and the stiffness of the band affects the amount the band can stretch (deformation). Note that the tension of a resistance band is equivalent to the product of its stiffness (k) and deformation (d), so tension = k X d. Increased stretching of the band results in a linear increase in the band's tension. Note that two similar bands can be different (3.2% to 5.2%), which will increase the amount of mean tension by 8% to 19%.

A resistance band can be attached to a barbell and then attached to a heavy dumbbell, or have a customized attachment on a squat rack. The resistance will be greatest when the band has the highest amount of tension. At the top position and the bottom position, there will be no resistance from the band because it is no longer stretched. Thus, the stretch load increases when the athlete is ascending from the bottom position and the load decreases as the athlete descends from the top position. Once the loads at the top and bottom positions are determined, those values are averaged. If an athlete wants to use a 5-RM load of 150 kg using bands, the average of bands at the two positions is subtracted from the original load on the bar. If an athlete is doing a bench press and the load at the bottom is 0 kg and the load at the top is 26.6 kg, the average is 13.3 kg. This average would be subtracted from the total weight on the bar (without bands), so the athlete would put between 136 kg and 137 kg on the bar, attach the bands, and complete the resistance exercise.

Nontraditional Implement-Training Methods

Strongman Training: Utilizes nontraditional implements such as tires, logs, weighted sleds, and stones. Research on the efficacy of strongman exercises is limited, but there is some evidence indicating that strongman exercises can be used as high-intensity training stimuli that increase blood lactate levels. The exercises have a greater amount of instability and are more challenging for the athletes than typical resistance-training exercises.

Tire Flipping

The dimensions of the tire must be considered to match the appropriate tire for each athlete. The tire should not be taller than the athlete when he or she is standing upright. As the height of the tire increases, so does the difficulty of flipping the tire. In addition to height, width of the tire needs to be considered. The tire should not be too narrow or wide for the athlete. Shorter athletes have difficulty flipping wider tires because of their short arm length. Taller athletes generally have difficulty with narrow tires because of arm length and depth requirements. Tire treads that are too worn can be difficult to grip while treads that are pronounced may contain debris or exposed metal that could cause an injury. There are three flipping techniques that can be employed in training. In the sumo style, the approach is characterized by a wide sumo deadlift stance with the arms positioned in a narrow grip. The athlete raises the tire to hip or chest height and then rotates his or her hands to a forward-pressing action that flips the tire. In the backlift style, athletes use a narrower stance (feet at hip-width) and flex the knees and hips to grab and pull the tire. This is similar to the motion for a deadlift. The athlete repositions his or her hands when tire is raised, allowing for a forward-pressing action that flips the tire. With the shoulders-against-the-tire technique, the athlete kneels behind the tire with the feet at hip-width with dorsiflexed ankles. The chin and shoulders are placed on the tire (similar to the position for a barbell front squat) with a supinated grip, using a wider width for a narrow tire and narrower width for a wide tire. The athlete raises his or her knees from the ground while on the balls of the feet. Most the athlete's weight is on the tire because the center of gravity shifts to the tire. The chest is then raised while the musculature of lower back contracts. To push the tire forward and up, the knees and hips are extended while the ankles plantarflex. The shoulders and hips rise simultaneously and the athlete takes two to three steps forward. When the tire is at hip height, one hip is flexed, the quadriceps hit the tire, and the athlete moves the hands into a pronated position. The feet move toward the tire while arms extend to push the tire over.

Log Lifting
The typical lifting movement is related to the movement in a power clean, although other movements (e.g., presses, rows, deadlifts, jerks, lunges, and squats) can be used. Logs are designed to be used with a mid-range pronated grip position. Logs can also have weight added to them but in most cases, the athlete is not able to lift as much as during a traditional resistance exercise. To date, no research has examined the efficacy of log lifting as a training method or determined how the training can be used for preparing athletes for the demands of sport.

Farmer's Walk
The athlete holds a static or variable load (e.g., water filled) at each side while walking forward. Unstable and awkward loads or resistances are thought to be useful for training because they require the athlete to engage the core. Although research is limited, Farmer's walks may facilitate the development of total-body anaerobic endurance, grip strength, and back endurance, although there is no research to date evaluating the safety of the exercise.

Kettlebell Training
A kettlebell is a weighted implement comprised of a ball with an attached handle that can be used a variety of exercises such as kettlebell swings, single leg Romanian deadlifts, and Sumo squats. Research has shown that kettlebells can be used to develop fitness. Kettlebell swings positively affect cardiovascular fitness, although to a lesser degree than treadmill running or other types of aerobic exercise. Kettlebells have been found to increase muscular strength levels. Six weeks of kettlebell training has been shown to improve vertical-jump performance and muscular strength, but these improvements are less than those achieved with traditional resistance-training exercises. Kettlebells are best used for general preparation exercises such as squats and bent-over rows, while more traditional modes of exercise are used to develop strength and enhance athletic performance. There are different types of kettlebells. Sport kettlebells are made of steel and all weights are the same size while cast-iron fitness kettlebells are various sizes depending on weight. To select the appropriate kettlebell, the handle size is based on the weight of cast-iron kettlebells, with increasing handle size corresponding to increasing weight. Polished steel handles should be chosen over painted handles because steel handles grip chalk better and do not get as slippery from sweat as painted handles.

Unilateral Training
Unilateral or bilateral training can be used for the upper or lower body. Unilateral exercises are often used to reduce an athlete's bilateral asymmetries when asymmetries exist between unilateral and bilateral movements. They are also used as part of rehabilitation programs. Bilateral movements have been shown to increase voluntary activation of the agonist muscle(s). This is known as bilateral facilitation and it is observed in trained athletes and stronger athletes. Athletes who are untrained, weaker, or injured should use unilateral training. However, trained athletes should avoid this training style.

Examples of lower-body unilateral exercises include:

- Step-ups
- Lunges
- Single-leg squats/ Bulgarian split squats

Plyometric Training

Explosive activities, such as plyometrics, use the stretch-shortening cycle (the fast lengthening and shortening of a muscle) to create muscle contractions. The stretch-shortening cycle involves an eccentric phase, amortization phase, and concentric phase. A muscle shortens in the concentric phase and lengthens in the eccentric phase. The amortization phase is the transition between the eccentric and concentric phases. Muscle spindles are essential to the stretch-reflex response because they are the primary proprioceptive structures in the muscle. Muscle spindles respond to eccentric muscle action. When muscles experience eccentric contractions during plyometric exercises, the muscles and surrounding tendons stretch and store energy. This musculotendinous unit where elastic energy is stored is called the series elastic component (SEC). The SEC works like a spring that returns the lengthened muscle to its shortened state during a concentric contraction. As the muscle shortens, energy is released. An athlete can use this energy to generate enough force to complete the plyometric exercises.

Lower-Body Plyometrics
Including lower-body plyometric exercises in an athlete's training program can improve sport performance by increasing the athlete's ability to produce greater force in a shorter period of time. Lower-body plyometric exercises are appropriate for almost every sport, including track and field events, sprinting, soccer, volleyball, football, baseball, basketball, cycling, distance running, and triathlons. Different sports require different movement patterns. Lateral and horizontal movements are used in baseball, football, and sprinting, while volleyball requires vertical and horizontal movements. Some sports like soccer and basketball require powerful and quick movements with changes in direction and planes. In addition to improving the force and velocity of movement, endurance athletes also benefit because lower-body plyometric training improves muscle efficiency by training muscles to produce more force using less energy. Lower-body plyometric exercises that can be included in an athlete's training program from lowest to highest intensity include jumps in place, standing jumps, multiple hops and jumps (also called countermovement jumps), bounds, box drills, and depth jumps. Training adaptations can be obtained over relatively short periods of time (six to ten weeks), but athletes can benefit from plyometric training throughout the macrocycle.

Upper-Body Plyometrics
Upper-body plyometric exercises use the same neuromuscular mechanisms as lower-body plyometric exercises to produce sports movements. Upper-body plyometric exercises should be included in training programs for athletes participating in sports that require fast and powerful upper-body movements. These sports include tennis, softball, golf, baseball, field throwing (e.g., shot put, discus, and javelin), lacrosse, swimming, and other sprint and endurance activities. Sports requiring tackling, catching, and holding off opponents can also benefit from upper-body plyometric training. Although upper-body plyometric exercises (e.g., medicine ball throwing and catching, and plyometric push-ups) are an essential training component for athletes requiring upper-body power, these exercises are not as commonly used as lower-body plyometric exercises.

Modifications for Performing Trunk Plyometrics

It is difficult to perform a true plyometric trunk exercise because the mechanical and neurophysiological mechanisms necessary for the stretch-shortening cycle may not be present. Although some elastic energy may be stored during plyometric trunk exercises, research suggests that the stretch reflex is not sufficiently involved for potentiated muscle-contraction activity to occur. The abdominal muscles are close to the spinal cord, which may result in shorter latencies for the abdominal stretch reflex. The large range of motion and time associated with the trunk movements inhibit the potentiation of the abdominal muscles. However, altering the exercise movements so that they are shorter and quicker may cause rapid eccentric muscle loading that elicits the stretch reflex and results in potentiated contraction of the muscle.

Frequency of Plyometric Training Activities

The frequency of plyometric training is primarily influenced by the athlete's sport, previous experience with plyometric training, the phase of training in a cycle or season, and the intensity and volume of daily workouts, including plyometrics, resistance training, sport practices, and aerobic training. For most sports, an athlete can perform one to three training sessions per week with forty-eight to seventy-two hours of recovery time in between plyometric training sessions. In order to determine plyometric training frequency, the strength and conditioning professional must evaluate the intensity of the plyometric exercises performed, the number of repetitions completed for each exercise, and the total volume of all other types of training. Because there is very limited research about the frequency of plyometric training, guidelines for the frequency of training do not exist.

Plyometric Training Volumes

Plyometric exercise volumes are commonly determined as the number of repetitions and sets that are completed during a single training session. Training volumes for lower-body plyometric exercises are expressed as the number of foot contacts during a session. For example, if an athlete is doing bounding exercises, volume may be expressed as a total distance covered. Training volume for upper-body plyometrics is typically expressed as the number of catches or throws during a training session. An athlete's level of plyometrics experience is used to provide a suggested training volume.

- Beginner: 80-100 repetitions per session
- Intermediate: 100-120 repetitions per session
- Advanced: 120-140 repetitions per session

Age Considerations and Possible Limitations for Plyometric Training Activities

A wide variety of ages – not just the elite adult athlete – can safely benefit from plyometric and plyometric-like exercises if appropriate guidelines are followed. This is particularly true for prepubescent and adolescent children who gain muscular power and bone strength from participating in an appropriately designed plyometric program. Young athletes who regularly participate in plyometric training gain enhanced neuromuscular control and performance, helping to prepare them for the demands of sport competitions and practices. Plyometric programs designed for children should focus on developing correct technique to ensure quality movements while performing the plyometric activities and should progress from simple to more difficult plyometric exercises. Among prepubescent athletes, depth jumps and high-intensity lower-body exercises are contraindicated because they can cause the epiphyseal growth plates to close prematurely, resulting in the stunting of limb growth. Adequate recovery time of two to three days should separate the plyometric training sessions for young athletes. Master athletes also benefit from plyometric training but the goals of the program and preexisting orthopedic and joint degeneration must be considered when designing the plyometric training program. With a few exceptions, the same general program development guidelines used for adult athletes can be used for developing training programs for older athletes. The program should not include more than five low-to-moderate intensity exercises, the volume should be lower, and there should be three to four recovery days between training sessions.

Speed/Sprint Training

Important Definitions
- Rate of Force Development (RFD): The change in force divided by the change in time; a sprinter wants to generate maximal force in minimal time.

- Impulse: The product of the time that force is applied to the ground and the amount of force applied.

- Momentum: The relationship between the mass of an object and the velocity of movement; an increased impulse (due to greater force generation) results in either an increase in momentum (acceleration or reacceleration) or a decrease in momentum (deceleration).

Methods for Improving Sprinting
Method #1: Sprinting
The best way to improve speed (i.e., running velocity) is to do maximum-velocity sprint training. Sprinting relies on an athlete's ability to produce high forces in a short period of time. Inclusion of maximum-velocity sprinting in long-term training plans can produce neurological adaptations that can improve RFD and impulse generation. Resisted and assisted sprint training techniques are commonly used to enhance force production or specific neuromuscular adaptations in order to enhance sprinting performance.

Resisted Sprint Training Techniques for Speed Development: Resisted sprint training techniques include modalities such as using harnesses for sled and parachute towing, uphill running, weighted vests, wind resistance, and sled pushing. The objectives of resisted sprint techniques are to enhance the acceleration phase biomechanics and to produce greater propulsive forces so that the athlete can cover longer distances faster. The strength and conditioning coach should be aware that loads used for training are sport-specific. Sprinters should use lighter loads (i.e., loads that do not decrease velocity by more than 10% to 12%) while field athletes who are exposed to external resistance may use loads that are 20% to 30% of the athlete's body weight.

Assisted Sprint Training Techniques for Speed Development: The goal of assisted sprint training techniques is to produce an overspeed effect that causes the athlete to run at a faster pace than normal. This increased pace supports adaptation of the athlete's neuromuscular system to contract at faster rates, thus allowing athletes to increase their stride rate and maximum sprint velocity. Assisted training techniques include pulling the athlete with cords (e.g., rope towing, elastic-band/surgical-tubing pulls), high-speed treadmill sprinting with a specialized treadmill, and downhill running. Strength and conditioning professionals should recognize that running mechanics can be difficult to regulate at high speeds. The maximum speed should be no greater than 110% of the athlete's known maximal speed.

If speed is too great, it can lead to the following issues:

- Rushing the stance phase, which lessens the time available to produce propulsive force production

- Increasing braking forces while being towed due to the athlete's inability to handle the increased velocity

- Exposure to significant eccentric forces during downhill running due to the modified mechanics of altered foot placement

Because assisted sprint training can have detrimental effects, it is critical to consider the athlete's biomechanics and training status when deciding whether to implement assisted sprinting techniques.

Method #2: Strength
Sprint speed is dependent upon the ability to produce large forces in a minimal period of time. Weight training plays a critical role when training sprint athletes. One issue that strength and conditioning professionals need to be aware of is the importance of being able to transfer the strength qualities from the weight room to the track. Making the movement pattern, RFD, peak force, and acceleration and velocity patterns in a weight-training program specific to the demands of the sport can facilitate this transfer of the training effect.

Method #3: Mobility
Mobility Training: Mobility (the athlete's ability to move a limb through a specific range of motion) and mobility training are part of dynamic flexibility training programs. Mobility and flexibility are both important components of correct agility and sprinting mechanics because maximum range of motion is needed to perform these activities. Common sprinting mechanics issues include improper arm swinging, premature upright posture, neck hyperextension, and bouncing. A strength and conditioning professional can correct these errors to improve mobility. Helping the athlete to lengthen the push-off and stride can help vertical bouncing; keeping a steady eye level can help premature upright posture; and keeping eyes focused on the ground will improve neck hyperextension. The recovery phase is key because the sprinter's body is aligned in a way that will enhance speed.

An athlete's speed and agility may also be limited by compromised joint mobility or flexibility. Joints with poor mobility and flexibility produce improper forces, reduce sprinting speed and agility capabilities, and increase the risk for injury. Optimal mobility and flexibility allow the athlete to have fluid movements, which can help to increase turnover rates during the phases of sprinting and agility activities. Strength and conditioning professionals need to be aware of an athlete's mobility or flexibility limitations so that they can design programs that will increase mobility and flexibility and enhance sprinting and agility. Assessing the athlete's muscular balance, activity levels, and range of motion can help identify issues that can be improved and corrected through a focused training program.

Mobility Drills: Dynamic stretching is sometimes referred to as mobility drills. Mobility drills emphasize sport-specific movement requirements instead of individual muscle movements. In addition to increasing range of motion, mobility drills are beneficial for pre-sport activity (i.e., training or competition) because they increase blood flow to muscle tissue, synovial fluid circulation to the joints, body temperature, and central nervous system activity. These physiological changes are consistent with those that occur when an athlete goes from a resting to an active state. Mobility drills are the ideal pre-activity stretching method because static stretching does not produce the aforementioned physiological changes and ballistic stretching is not as safe as mobility drills. Mobility drills for swimmers may include

131

shoulder raises and arm swings, while drills for runners may include walking knee lifts, inverted hamstring stretches, and lunge walks.

Agility Training

Agility is a multicomponent skill in response to a sport-specific stimulus. It includes the ability to change direction, velocity, or mode in response to a stimulus. Agility also requires perceptual-cognitive skills such as pattern recognition of players on a playing field, visual scanning, anticipation, accuracy, and reaction time.

Reaction time allows the athlete to make quick decisions based on how the nervous system and muscular system react to a stimulus. Because an athlete's ability to process a stimulus cannot be trained, improvements to reaction time will be small regardless of the training. Also, faster reaction times only result in better decision-making but do not affect performance in explosive activities.

Agility-drill types include continuous drills, discrete drills, and serial drills. Continuous drills have no beginning or end and they are helpful for improving running and jumping. Discrete drills help to develop movement patterns and improve an athlete's strength and power. Serial drills are sport specific and combine continuous and discrete drills. Together, these drill types can improve strength, change-of-direction (COD) ability, and perceptual-cognitive ability.

<u>Methods for Developing Agility</u>
Method #1: Strength
Dynamic Strength: This is the base strength that is needed for all other strength training. Dynamic strength can help provide mobility during bodyweight-only and loaded training. Examples of dynamic strength exercises for athletes include calisthenics, squats, pulls, and change-of-direction drills.

Eccentric Strength: Developing eccentric strength improves the ability to effectively absorb load during the brake phase of a COD. Examples of eccentric strength exercises for athletes include drop landings, receiving strength required during catch phase of Olympic lifts, accentuated eccentric training, and deceleration drills (high velocity, various angles).

Multidirectional Strength: This type of strength improves the athlete's ability to hold the body position during movement demands. Examples of such exercises include lunges, Z-drills, unilateral lifts, high-velocity COD drills, and cutting-angle COD drills.

Reactive Strength: Having reactive strength enhances the athlete's ability to transfer from high eccentric load to concentric explosiveness. Examples of reactive strength exercises include plyometrics, drop jumps, and loaded jumps.

Concentric Explosive Strength: Athletes need concentric explosive strength to reaccelerate after the breaking phase. This type of strength is required for the maintenance of a strong position through the transition phase of COD and agility. Example exercises include box jumps, acceleration drills, loaded squat jumps, sled pushes, and Olympic lifts.

Method #2: COD Ability

Closed-skill COD drills progress similarly to the progression plyometric exercises based on the difficulty and intensity of each drill. The following list provides examples of progressing deceleration drills for athletes at various levels:

- Beginner Level: The athlete would start with forward deceleration drills and progress with a higher entry velocity or shorter stopping distance.

- Intermediate Level: The athlete would do lateral deceleration drills and progress with a higher entry velocity or shorter stopping distance.

- Advanced Level: The athlete would do a drill requiring deceleration to reacceleration in forward and lateral directions.

Method #3: Perceptual-Cognitive Ability

Perceptual-cognitive ability can be trained by increasing the demands of the task in order to improve performance. Within-sport skills include visual scanning and pattern recognition. Drills to improve agility focus on improving accuracy, anticipation, and decision-making time. The following list provides examples of progressing agility activities to improve perceptual-cognitive abilities for athletes at various levels:

- Beginner Level: Closed-skill COD drills with an added perceptual-cognitive element can become agility drills by including a generic stimulus such as a coach's instruction, flashing light, or whistle blow.

- Advanced Level: Drills that use sport-specific stimuli (e.g., evasive drills, small-sided games) have been shown to have a greater affect on performance.

- Note: By progressively increasing the time (temporal) or spatial stress on the athlete, generic and specific stimuli within an agility skill can both be made more difficult.

Aerobic Training

Pace/Tempo Training Method

This training method is a type of aerobic endurance training that utilizes an intensity consistent with or slightly higher than race or competition intensity. The goal of pace/tempo training is to replicate the pattern of muscle fiber recruitment and physiological stress during competition in order to improve running economy, increase aerobic- and anaerobic-energy production, and increase lactate threshold. The intensity in this type of training – sometimes called threshold training or aerobic-anaerobic interval training – corresponds to the lactate threshold and improves the aerobic- and anaerobic-energy systems, which are both active during a race. Pace/tempo training can either be steady or intermittent. Steady training consists of a twenty- to thirty-minute bout of continuous training at the athlete's lactate threshold. During exercise, muscle cells release lactate into the blood. Resting levels of blood lactate range between 0.8 nM (nanomolar) and 1.5 nM and lactate levels can be greater than 18 nM during intense exercise. The lactate threshold is the amount of work (i.e., percentage of VO_2 max) that causes blood lactate concentrations to increase above resting levels. In aerobic training, lactate threshold can refer to the speed of movement or exercise intensity that is associated with a specific concentration of lactate in the blood. When athletes exceed their lactate threshold during exercise, they experience substantial physical and mental fatigue. Intermittent training is similar to the steady pace/tempo approach, except that the work intervals are separated by short recovery periods. When doing pace/tempo training, it is important that the work is done at the prescribed intensity. Athletes should avoid working at a more intense pace. This type of training is generally done one to two times per week for twenty to thirty minutes, at the athlete's normal race pace.

Long, Slow Distance (LSD) Running

LSD training is usually done one to two times per week at an intensity of approximately 70% VO_2 max and 80% of maximal heart rate. This type of training is slower than race pace. The distance covered should be longer than the race distance and the training duration should be thirty minutes to two hours. Several physiological adaptations arise from LSD, including improved thermoregulation, cardiovascular function, mitochondrial energy production, and use of fat as energy. Lactate threshold may also increase as these adaptations make clearing lactate from the blood easier. Too much LSD can be detrimental to race performance, because neuromuscular adaptations may be made to a running intensity that is significantly lower than that required during a race.

Fartlek Training

Fartlek literally means "speed play." It combines several types of endurance training and can be used for runners, swimmers, and cyclists. Fartlek training involves low-intensity exercise (approximately 70% VO_2 max) with short bursts of high-intensity (85% to 95% VO_2 max) exercise at more irregular points, lengths, and speeds than in interval training. Fartlek training can provide an opportunity for athletes to challenge themselves on a weekly basis and help relieve the monotony of a single type of training session. It is best used during periods of heavy training leading up to an event. This type of training challenges all body systems and can improve VO_2 max, lactate threshold, energy consumption, and exercise economy. Fartlek training is generally done once per week for twenty to sixty minutes. The intensity varies from LSD to pace/tempo.

High-Intensity Interval Training (HIIT)

This training uses repeated high-intensity ($\geq$90% VO_2 max) exercise bouts with rest periods in between. Depending on the desired training response, short exercise bouts of forty-five seconds or less or long bouts of two to four minutes can be used. As the duration of the high-intensity exercise gets longer, blood lactate levels will increase because energy will come from anaerobic glycolysis. The length of the rest periods between the intervals is important. Rest periods that are too short will not allow the athlete to recover enough to put forth the required effort necessary to complete the remaining high-intensity bouts. If the rest period is too long, the athlete's body may not require energy from anaerobic glycolysis and the training response will not occur. An example of appropriate work-to-rest time periods would be two to three minutes of high-intensity exercise followed by a rest period of two minutes. Running economy and speed may be improved by HIIT. This type of training is typically done once per week.

Flexibility Training

Flexibility consists of static and dynamic components and is a measure of range of motion (ROM). ROM is the degree of movement that occurs at a joint.

Static flexibility is the amount of movement around a joint during a passive movement. Static flexibility is not dependent on voluntary movement. A partner, gravity, or a machine provides the force required for the stretch.

Dynamic flexibility is the ROM during active movements requiring voluntary muscle activity. In general, dynamic ROM is greater than static ROM.

For flexibility and performance, the type of sport-specific movements that athletes must perform dictates the level of flexibility they need. The strength and conditioning professional needs to base an athlete's flexibility training on the requirements of the sport, as well as the force patterns required through the ROM. Injury risk may increase if an athlete is unable to obtain the level of flexibility required by the sport. Likewise, hyperflexibility can also increase the risk for injury.

Factors affecting flexibility include:

- Joint Structure: The type and shape of the joint (i.e., ball-and-socket, ellipsoidal, hinge) and its surrounding tissue affect its ROM.

- Muscle and Connective Tissue: Many body tissues (e.g., tendons, muscle, fascial sheaths, skin, joint capsules, and ligaments) can limit ROM. Stretching takes advantage of the plasticity and elasticity of connective tissues and can affect ROM.

- Muscle Bulk: ROM can be negatively affected by substantial muscle bulk. The specific requirements of the sport (e.g., large muscles versus joint mobility) should be considered when determining a flexibility program for an athlete.

- Neural Control: ROM is controlled by the central and peripheral nervous systems, so an effective flexibility program needs to affect both systems.

- Stretch Tolerance: How well athletes can tolerate the discomfort of stretching influences their ROM. Athletes with a greater stretch tolerance generally have a greater ROM.

- Resistance Training: Heavy resistance training can decrease ROM; however, an appropriately planned resistance-training program can actually increase ROM. Increased ROM can enhance the development of force capacity.

- Activity Level: Active individuals are generally more flexible than inactive individuals, particularly if the activity includes flexibility exercises.

- Age and Sex: Young people are generally more flexible than older people, and women are generally more flexible than men.

Combining Various Training Methods/Modes to Reach a Goal or Outcome

Muscular Endurance can be improved through resistance and circuit training.

Hypertrophy can result from resistance training. Research indicates performing ≥3 exercises per muscle group will optimize increases in muscle size.

Strength gains can be achieved through resistance, bodyweight, and Strongman training.

Power improves via complex training, which combines heavy resistance training and plyometric exercises with the goal of enhancing short-term power output. Complex training uses a training stimulus that couples a heavy load (i.e., resistance exercise) with a light load (i.e., plyometric exercise) in order to optimize force and power production beyond that which can be achieved with either exercise alone. The enhanced force and power production is a result of a phenomenon call post-activation potentiation (PAP). The principle behind PAP is that heavy loading causes significant stimulation of the central nervous system, which leads to greater motor-unit recruitment and force. The increased muscle activation resulting from the heavy load produces a faster contraction rate. By pairing a high-intensity resistance exercise set with a biomechanically similar plyometric exercise set, the resulting PAP increases force development and maximizes the production of explosive power for athletic performance. An example of complex training is a set of two to three back squats (85% to 90%) followed by three to five vertical jumps to maximal height, with a rest period of three minutes between the two exercises. Examples of other complex training sets are bench press followed by plyometric push-up and barbell lunge followed by single-leg hops.

Aerobic Endurance can be improved by combining resistance training with aerobic endurance training. Such training will provide short-term exercise performance improvements and increased strength that can help with hill climbing, the final sprint of an endurance competition, and catching up to competitors when there are breakaway groups. Resistance training can also be beneficial for faster recovery from injuries and the prevention of overuse injuries and muscle imbalances. Plyometric training can also progress aerobic endurance. Many sports, such as soccer and tennis, have both a power (anaerobic) and aerobic component. Performing plyometric exercises before aerobic endurance training can help to minimize the detrimental effect that aerobic training can have on power production. Altitude training can also be beneficial. Increased altitude causes a reduction in the partial pressure of oxygen due to drops in atmospheric pressure, which detrimentally affects gas exchange in the lungs. The body attempts to compensate for the reduced partial pressure with a number of physiological changes. It takes twelve to fourteen days for the body to acclimatize to altitude up to 2,300 meters. Some athletes train at altitude or attempt to get the benefits of altitude training by using the "live high, train low" (LHTL) method. This requires the athlete to live at moderate altitudes (2,000 to 3,000 meters) and train at sea level. Living at high altitude results in metabolic and hematological adaptations that can provide ergogenic benefits by enhancing neuromuscular development during lower-altitude training. Any of the various types of aerobic training (e.g., LSD, pace/tempo, interval, HIIT, or Fartlek training) can be completed as part of altitude training.

Selecting Exercises

<u>Exercises Specific to the Movement Patterns of a Particular Sport</u>
Ball Dribbling and Passing
Exercises and muscles used for these movements include:

- Dumbbell Bench Press: Pectoralis major, anterior deltoids, triceps brachii
- Triceps Pushdown: Triceps brachii
- Hammer Curl: Brachialis, biceps brachii, brachioradialis
- Close-Grip Bench Press: Sternal pectoralis major, anterior deltoid, clavicular pectoralis major, triceps brachii
- Reverse Curl: Brachioradialis, brachialis, biceps brachii

Freestyle Swimming (including starts and turns)
Exercises and muscles used for these movements include:

- Pull-Up: Lower and middle trapezius, biceps brachii, pectoralis minor, teres major, brachialis, rhomboids, brachioradialis, levator scapulae, latissimus dorsi, teres minor, infraspinatus, posterior deltoid

- Forward Step Lunge: Biceps femoris, rectus femoris, gluteus maximus, iliopsoas, semimembranosus, vastus medialis, semitendinosus, vastus lateralis, vastus intermedius

- Lateral Shoulder Raise: Deltoids

- Upright Row: Deltoids, upper trapezius

- Barbell Pullover: Rhomboids, latissimus dorsi, posterior deltoid, sternal pectoralis major, teres major, pectoralis minor, levator scapulae, long head triceps

- Single-Leg Squat: Quadriceps, gluteus maximus, adductor magnus, soleus, erector spinae

Running, Sprinting
Exercises and muscles used for these movements include:

- Clean: Gluteus maximus, gastrocnemius, semimembranosus, semitendinosus, trapezius, biceps femoris, deltoids, vastus lateralis, vastus medialis, vastus intermedius, soleus, rectus femoris

- Snatch: Deltoids, semimembranosus, soleus, semitendinosus, trapezius, vastus lateralis, vastus intermedius, gastrocnemius, vastus medialis, biceps femoris, rectus femoris, gluteus maximus

- Front Squat: Biceps femoris, gluteus maximus, rectus femoris, semimembranosus, vastus lateralis, vastus intermedius, semitendinosus, vastus medialis

- Forward Step Lunge: Iliopsoas, biceps femoris, vastus lateralis, semimembranosus, gluteus maximus, semitendinosus, vastus intermedius, rectus femoris, vastus medialis

- Step-Up: Vastus medialis, gluteus maximus, vastus lateralis, semimembranosus, biceps femoris, semitendinosus, rectus femoris, vastus intermedius

- Leg (Knee) Curl: Semimembranosus, biceps femoris, semitendinosus

- Leg (Knee) Extension: Vastus medialis, rectus femoris, vastus intermedius, vastus lateralis

Exercises Based on the Type/Number of Involved Muscle Group(s)
Core Exercises
Also called multi-joint exercises, core exercises involve two or more primary joints and recruit one or more large muscle areas (e.g., shoulder, thigh, back, etc.). Multi-joint exercises stimulate muscles the most because they recruit all of the large muscle groups associated with the involved joints. As a result, they allow for the greatest amount of loading during resistance training. These exercises should be used for athletes who have a limited amount of time to train.

Examples:

- Bench Press: Sternal pectoralis major, clavicular pectoralis major, anterior deltoids, triceps brachii

- Front Squat: Biceps femoris, gluteus maximus, rectus femoris, vastus intermedius, semimembranosus, vastus lateralis, semitendinosus, vastus medialis

- Deadlift: Vastus intermedius, gluteus maximus, vastus lateralis, biceps femoris, semimembranosus, rectus femoris, semitendinosus, vastus medialis

Structural Exercises:
Structural exercises are core exercises that specifically emphasize loading the spine. Loading of the spine can be direct (e.g., back squat) or indirect (e.g., power clean). A structural exercise requires the muscular stabilization of posture during the lifting movement. For example, during a back squat the athlete maintains a rigid torso and a neutral spine. These types of exercises should be the basis of training programs.

Examples:

- Power Clean (all body, power/structural): Deltoids, soleus, semimembranosus, rectus femoris, semitendinosus, vastus lateralis, biceps femoris, vastus intermedius, trapezius, vastus medialis, gluteus maximus, gastrocnemius

- Back Squat: Vastus lateralis, vastus intermedius, semimembranosus, gluteus maximus, semitendinosus, rectus femoris, vastus medialis, biceps femoris

Power Exercises:
Power exercises are structural exercises that are performed very quickly or explosively. The strength and conditioning professional needs to assess the athlete's sport-specific training needs in order to determine if power exercises should be prescribed.

Examples:

- Push Press (all body, power): Deltoids, soleus, gluteus maximus, semimembranosus, vastus medialis, vastus intermedius, semitendinosus, vastus lateralis, rectus femoris, gastrocnemius, biceps femoris, trapezius

- Push Jerk (all body, power): Semitendinosus, gluteus maximus, semimembranosus, deltoids, rectus femoris, vastus lateralis, trapezius, vastus intermedius, biceps femoris, soleus, gastrocnemius, vastus medialis

- Clean: Vastus medialis, gluteus maximus, soleus, semimembranosus, gastrocnemius, vastus intermedius, biceps femoris, vastus lateralis, rectus femoris, trapezius, semitendinosus, deltoids

- Snatch (all body, power): Trapezius, soleus, gluteus maximus, vastus lateralis, semitendinosus, gastrocnemius, biceps femoris, vastus intermedius, vastus medialis, rectus femoris, semimembranosus, deltoids

Assistance Exercises:

Also called single-joint exercises, assistance exercises involve one primary joint and recruit smaller muscle areas (e.g., forearm, calf, lower back, anterior lower leg, etc.).

Examples:

- Abdominal Crunch (abdomen): Rectus abdominis
- Standing Calf-Raise Machine: Gastrocnemius, soleus
- Wrist Curl (forearms): Flexor carpi ulnaris, flexor carpi radialis, palmaris longus
- Lateral Shoulder Raise (shoulders): Deltoids
- Bent-Over Row (upper back): Middle trapezius, latissimus dorsi, posterior deltoids, rhomboids, teres major
- Lying Triceps Extensions (posterior upper arm): Triceps brachii
- Stiff-Leg Deadlift (posterior hip and thigh): Semimembranosus, gluteus maximus, biceps femoris, erector spinae, semitendinosus
- Hammer Curl (biceps): Brachialis, biceps brachii, brachioradialis
- Example of changing an exercise to change the muscles used (wrist) include:

  o Wrist Extensions (pronated grip on the bar): Extensor carpi radialis brevis and longus, extensor carpi ulnaris

  o Wrist Curl (supinated grip on the bar): Palmaris longus, flexor carpi ulnaris, flexor carpi radialis

Exercises Based on the Type of Kinetic Chain Movement
Open Kinetic Chain (OKC) Movements

OKC exercises are performed when the athlete's hands or feet are not in contact with a surface (i.e., the hands or feet are not fixed). OKC exercises for the lower extremity include knee-extension and leg-curl exercises. Examples of upper-extremity OKC exercises include triceps pushdowns, bicep curls, and wrist curls. OKC exercises allow for greater focus to be placed on specific joints or muscles.

Closed Kinetic Chain (CKC) Movements

CKC exercises are performed with the extremity in continual contact with a surface (e.g., feet on the ground or hands on a machine handle). The hands or feet do not move during the exercise. Examples of lower-extremity CKC exercises are squats, lunges, and leg presses. Examples of upper-extremity CKC exercises are pull-ups and push-ups. CKC exercises allow for increased joint stability and functional movement patterns.

Exercises to Minimize Injury Potential
Muscle Balance

Resistance-training programs designed for any sport should ensure that there is a balance in exercises across opposing muscle groups. Disparities in the strength of agonist and antagonist muscles can result in an increased risk of injury. For example, if the hamstrings are weaker than the quadriceps, then it is important to add hamstring exercises to the training program in order to address the muscle imbalance. Addressing muscle imbalance involves improving the *strength ratios* in antagonist muscle groups rather than making opposing muscle groups equally strong. One example of muscle balance is a 3:4 strength ratio between hamstrings and quadriceps.

Alternation of Upper- and Lower-Body Exercises
The alternation of upper- and lower-body resistance exercises during a training session increases recovery between exercises by maximizing the length of rest periods. Alternating exercises is beneficial for untrained athletes who may find doing multiple upper- or lower-body exercises in a row too strenuous.

Order of Resistance Exercises
The order of resistance exercises during a session should be power exercises, followed by core exercises, and then assistance exercises. Power exercises require the most skill and concentration and are detrimentally affected by fatigue. Fatigue can result in poor technique, which can increase the risk of injury.

Split Routine
Intermediate and advanced athletes may use a split routine where they focus on training different muscle groups on different days. This format allows athletes to do resistance training almost every day. Although training daily goes against the recommended one to three days of rest between resistance-training sessions, sessions focus on specific muscle groups so there is adequate recovery time between sessions that train the same groups of muscles. Adequate recovery time decreases the risk of overstressing the muscles and potentially increasing the risk of injury.

Flexibility
Athletes that do not have the level of flexibility required for their sport or have too much flexibility are at an increased risk of injury. Flexibility training can help to increase an athlete's ROM during sport-related movements. Hyperflexibility will require the strength and conditioning professional to take a close look at the athlete's resistance and flexibility programs to determine appropriate changes aimed at decreasing ROM. Increasing muscle bulk, heavy resistance training, and reducing flexibility exercises may help an athlete to minimize their hyperflexibility.

Exercises to Promote Recovery
A recovery exercise is any exercise that avoids high muscular or nervous stress while, at the same time, promoting movement and restoration. Recovery exercises help with the removal of metabolic waste and byproducts while maintaining blood flow to the exercised muscles. This helps to optimize the repair of the exercised muscles, facilitating recovery and restoration. Recovery exercises are commonly done at the end of the resistance-training session or during a separate session within the microcycle. Examples of recovery exercises include low-intensity aerobic exercise or lightly loaded resistance exercises.

Principles of Exercise Order

Order of Exercises Based on the Training Goal
Exercise order is the sequence of resistance exercises that are performed during one training session. There are numerous approaches for ordering exercises. Four common approaches are as follows:

- Power, then other core, then assistance exercises
- Alternated upper- and lower-body exercises
- Alternated "push" and "pull" exercises
- Supersets and compound sets

The strength and conditioning professional needs to consider how one resistance exercise affects the effort and technical quality of the subsequent exercise. It is critical that the need for technique and effort are considered in ordering resistance exercise because fatigue can cause athletes to use poor technique, thus increasing the risk for injury.

Variations in Exercise Orders
Power, Other Core, Assistance Exercises
Training sessions typically order the exercises from the most metabolically demanding and technical (i.e., power exercises) to the least demanding exercises (i.e., core and assistance exercises). For example, Olympic lifts are the most demanding power exercises because they place large metabolic demands on the athlete's body, require excellent technique and concentration, and are the most affected by fatigue. Accordingly, power exercises would be completed first during a training session. Non-power core exercises (i.e., multi-joint exercises) are completed next because they require quality technique, load the spine, and place large metabolic demands on the athlete's body. Finally, assistance or single-joint exercises are performed last because they are less technical and the least demanding resistance exercises. The strength and conditioning professional must consider both the technique and effort required when ordering resistance exercises because fatigue can cause athletes to use poor technique and increase their risk for injury.

Alternated Upper- and Lower-Body Exercises
Alternating upper- and lower-body resistance exercises allows for greater recovery between exercises. This training order is useful when training time is limited, because it minimizes the rest needed between exercises while maximizing the rest for the upper- and lower body between sets. When minimal rest is provided between sets, the method is called circuit training. Because circuit training requires an athlete to train with minimal rest between sets, this training style helps to improve mental focus. Also, the lack of rest requires the athlete to perform more exercises in a shorter period of time, and therefore helps to reduce body fat by imposing significant metabolic demands on the athlete.

Alternating "Push" and "Pull' Exercises
This variation alternates between pushing resistance exercises, such as shoulder presses or triceps extensions, with pulling exercises, such as bent-over rows and biceps curls. Alternating push and pull exercises improves recovery and recruitment between the exercises by ensuring that the same muscle group is not used in two consecutive exercises. Examples of push-pull exercise arrangements for the lower body include back squat (push) and leg (knee) curl (pull) and leg press (push) and stiff-leg deadlift (pull). Circuit training often uses alternating push and pull exercises. This ordering method can be used with athletes starting or returning to resistance exercise training.

Supersets
A superset is the performance of two resistance exercises sequentially. The first exercise stresses an agonist muscle or muscle groups and the second exercises stresses the antagonist muscle or muscle group. An example of a superset is ten repetitions of triceps pushdown followed immediately by ten repetitions of barbell biceps curls. Supersets efficiently use training time but may not be appropriate for unconditioned athletes or those needing significant training instruction.

Compound Sets
A compound set is the performance of two different resistance exercises in a row in order to stress the same muscle or the muscle groups. For example, a set of barbell biceps curls is followed immediately by dumbbell hammer curls. Compound sets are time-efficient and demanding, causing greater stress to the muscles. This type of training is not appropriate for unconditioned athletes.

<u>Variations in Exercise Modes</u>

Warm-Ups are usually ten to twenty minutes and consist of two specific periods or may be structured based on the raise, activate and mobilize, and potentiate (RAMP) protocol. The general warm-up period is five minutes of slow aerobic activity (e.g., jogging) followed by general stretching that focuses on ROM of the upcoming activities. This is followed by the specific warm-up period, which consists of movements that replicate those required for the upcoming activity. The RAMP Protocol consists of the following:

- Raise: Phase 1 of the protocol consists of activities that raise various physiological parameters like heart and respiration rates, body temperature, and blood flow. The activities simulate movement activities associated with the upcoming activity or develop skill patterns required for the specific sport.

- Activate and Mobilize: Phase 2 of the protocol focuses on mobility and may include dynamic stretching and mobility exercises.

- Potentiation: Phase 3 of the protocol is sport specific, with a focus on progressing the intensity of the activity to the intensity required for the training or competition.

- Note: This is followed by the planned workout, which may include resistance training, plyometrics, speed and agility, aerobic endurance, etc.

Explosive Training can include power exercises (structural exercises performed very fast) and various - plyometric exercises (e.g., box jumps, drop jumps, loaded jumps).

Strength Training can include the use of free weights, resistance machines, bodyweight, variable-resistance training methods (e.g., chain-supplemented exercises and resistance-band exercises), Strongman training (e.g., tire flipping, log lifting, farmer's walk), and kettlebell training.

Cooldown: This is a period of low-intensity exercise such as stretching that allows the body's physiological parameters to return to their normal levels.

Energy-System Training Prioritization
As mentioned, specific types of training can affect the phosphagen system, glycolytic system, and oxidative system in various ways. Carbohydrates, fats, and proteins can be metabolized for energy, but carbohydrates are the only macronutrient that can be metabolized without oxygen.

- Phosphagen System: The phosphagen system provides energy via anaerobic metabolism for brief, high-intensity activities (i.e., up to six seconds of extremely high-intensity exercise or six to thirty seconds of very high-intensity exercise). Modes of exercise that can be used to train the phosphagen system include doing resistance exercises in which each set has a low number of repetitions, sprinting less than 200 meters, and performing some types of plyometrics. To improve the phosphagen system's energy production, work-to-rest ratios for training should be between 1:12 and 1:20.

- Glycolytic System: The glycolytic system provides energy during moderate- to high-intensity and short- to medium-duration activities (i.e., thirty seconds to two minutes of high-intensity exercise or two to three minutes of moderate-intensity exercise). Glycolysis provides energy by breaking down muscle glycogen or blood glucose. Modes of exercise that can be used to train the glycolytic system include sprinting for 200 meters to 800 meters, doing high-intensity interval training, and performing some types of plyometrics. To improve the glycolytic system's energy production, work-to-rest ratios for training should be between 1:3 and 1:5.

- Oxidative (aerobic) System: This system is the primary source of energy during low-intensity and long-duration exercise (i.e., more than three minutes). The oxidative system uses carbohydrates (glucose and glycogen) and fats (triglycerides) to produce energy. Aerobic exercise at low-to-moderate intensities can be used to train the aerobic system. To improve the oxidative system's energy production, work-to-rest ratios for training should be 1:1 to 1:3.

Methods for Assigning an Exercise Load or Exercise Heart Rate

Exercise Loads

Repetition Maximum (RM): The repetition maximum (RM) is one of the critical components in designing a resistance-training program, and it is defined as the most weight that can be lifted for a specific number or repetitions. For example, if an athlete can complete six repetitions of the leg press using 100 lbs, the 6-RM is 100 lbs. The RM provides the strength and conditioning professional with information about the maximum number of repetitions that can be completed at a specific percentage of the 1-RM, which is then used to prescribe loading parameters. The RM provides the number of repetitions that can be completed using a specific weight, whereas the 1-RM requires calculations to be made to determine the percentage of the load to be used. The 1-RM may provide misleading information for some athletes because they can perform a 1-RM better (i.e., the athlete has a higher percentage of fast-twitch muscle fibers) or worse (i.e., the athlete has higher percentage of slow-twitch muscle fibers) than an RM. When possible, it is best to rely on the RM to determine training loads to ensure that the athlete is using the most accurate load.

1-RM: The one-repetition maximum (1-RM) is another critical component in designing a resistance-training program and is defined as the maximum amount of weight that an athlete can lift for only one repetition while maintaining correct technique. Assessment of an athlete's 1-RM for power and structural movements provides the strength and conditioning professional with information that will be used to determine training loads. Note that load is often discussed as the weight associated with a specific percentage of a 1-RM. The 1-RM will be used to establish the load parameters for the resistance training that will be used throughout the training program (i.e., load volumes used for single-training sessions and training weeks), as well as the purpose and goals of the specific training segment. It will be necessary for the strength and conditioning professional to reassess the 1-RM at the end of the training segment in order to evaluate improvements that accrued during the segment and to plan the components (i.e., load parameters, purpose, and goals) of the next training segment.

Exercise RPE

Assessing how hard athletes are working during a training session is critical to ensure that they are putting in appropriate amounts of effort. Asking the athletes how they feel is often not sufficient because the response is subjective with no way to adequately judge the intensity of the work. Numerous methods exist to help quantify the intensity level of an athlete's work during training. Ratings of perceived exertion (RPE) can be assessed using the BORG RPE scale. The original 15-point scale ranges from 6 (no exertion at all) to 20 (maximal exertion) while the revised 10-point scale ranges from 0 (very easy) to 10 (maximum effort). Importantly, both forms of the RPE scale provide the athlete with the ability to quantify perceived exertion. In general, the 15-point scale may be easiest for athletes to use, particularly if training sessions are based on training at a specific percentage of maximum heart rate or VO_2 max. There is a strong correlation between athletes' RPE score multiplied by 10 and their actual heart rate during exercise. For example, an RPE of 14 corresponds to an expected heart rate during exercise of 140 beats per minute. Note that RPE is the preferred method for evaluating exercise intensity among individuals that have conditions or take medications that affect their heart rate or pulse. The Borg RPE scale may be one of the easiest methods to communicate workout intensity levels. This scale is also a cost-friendly option, because it can be used without having to buy heart-rate monitors or other types of assessment systems. The table below depicts how the Borg RPE scale, the revised-RPE scale, percentage of maximum heart rate (i.e., intensity), and exercise type are related.

How Borg RPE Scales, Type of Exercise, and Percentage of Maximum Heart Rate Are Related

BORG RPE SCALE	BORG REVISED-RPE SCALE	EXERCISE TYPE	PERCENT OF MAXIMUM HEART RATE
6	0	WARM-UP	50%-60%
7			
8	1		
9			
10	2	RECOVERY	60%-70%
11			
12	3		
13		AEROBIC	70%-80%
14	4		
15	5	ANAEROBIC	80%-90%
16	6		
17	7	VO$_2$ max	90%-100%
18	8		
19	9		
20	10		

Exercise Heart Rate

Maximal Heart Rate (MHR): MHR refers to the highest heart rate achieved during a maximal-exercise (VO$_2$ max) test. This is the preferred method for determining exercise intensities that are associated with a specific percentage of MHR because it is based on the most accurate MHR data.

Age-Predicted Maximal Heart Rate (APMHR): If it is not possible to conduct a VO$_2$ max test to obtain an athlete's MHR, alternative methods, such as APMHR, may be used. The APMHR is calculated using a simple formula (220 - athlete's chronological age = predicted MHR). This is a general estimation that does not take into account actual heart-rate capacity, so the calculated predicted MHR may be higher or lower than the actual MHR. APMHR for a 20-year old male is calculated as APMHR: 220 − 20 = 200 beats/min. If this athlete wants to exercise at 70% intensity, his target heart rate would be calculated as follows: 200 beats/min x .70 = 140 beats/min.

Karvonen Method: The Karvonen method provides a better estimate of target heart rate because it accounts for the athlete's resting heart rate (RHR), an indicator of fitness level. The Karvonen method uses the following formula:

$$\text{Target Heart Rate} = \big((\text{APMHR} - \text{RHR}) \times \% \text{ intensity}\big) + \text{RHR}$$

For example, the target heart rate (also known as the percentage of MHR) is calculated for a 20-year-old athlete with a RHR of 50 beats/minute and a goal training intensity of 70% by first using the APMHR formula to calculate the estimated maximal heart rate: 220 - 20 = 200 beats/min. Then the RHR is subtracted from this value (200 - 50 = 150 beats/min). From here, the desired intensity is factored in by multiplying ((APMHR - RHR) x % intensity), which in this case is (150 beats/min x .70) = 105 beats/min. In the last step, target heart rate is calculated by adding RHR back to this value: 105 beats/min + 50 beats/min (RHR) = 155 beats/min.

Functional Capacity (heart-rate reserve, or HRR): Prescribing aerobic-exercise intensity using heart rate is very common because of the close relationship between an athlete's heart rate and oxygen consumption. Functional capacity is also known as HRR, and it is the difference between the MHR and RHR (MHR - RHR). HRR is the most accurate method for prescribing and adjusting aerobic-training intensity because it takes advantage of the relationship between heart rate and oxygen consumption and HRR accounts for physiological adaptation to aerobic-exercise training by taking RHR into consideration.

RHR can decrease over time in response to training. As an athlete's RHR decreases, HRR increases. The increase in HRR allows the athlete to exercise longer at a given intensity while experiencing less fatigue. The most accurate way to assess functional capacity is to do a laboratory-based VO_2 max test. This assessment is often not available to strength and conditioning professionals, so an alternative method – such as APMHR – can be used to prescribe training intensity.

Lactate
Lactate Threshold: Some research suggests that an athlete's lactate threshold may be a better indicator of aerobic capacity than VO_2 max. The strength and conditioning professional can work to increase an athlete's lactate threshold, thus allowing the athlete to work harder and longer. Increasing lactate threshold can improve performance and enhance recovery from competition and training, ultimately resulting in the athlete being able to sustain higher work rates in competitions.

Maximal-Lactate Steady State: Maximal-lactate steady state is defined as the exercise intensity at which the maximal amount of lactate produced by the muscles is equivalent to the maximum amount of lactate that can be removed from the body. This state reflects the highest exercise intensity that an athlete can sustain before quickly becoming fatigued when the lactate threshold is crossed. The maximal-lactate steady state provides information about the exercise intensity level and duration that allows the athlete to maintain the balance between lactate production and clearing. This information can be used for designing endurance-training programs in which the athlete must exceed the lactate threshold in order to increase the maximal-lactate steady state and improve endurance performance.

Load or Exercise Heart Rate Based on the Training Goal

Load-Based Training for Resistance Exercise
Recommended Percentage of 1-RM Load Based on Training Goals:

- Muscular Endurance: ≤ 67%
- Hypertrophy: 67% to 85%
- Strength: ≥ 85%
- Power, Single Effort (e.g., long jump, discus): 80% to 90%
- Power, Multiple Effort (e.g., volleyball, basketball): 75% to 85%

Aerobic Endurance and Heart Rate for Training Goals

Aerobic endurance-training programs are generally designed to improve maximal aerobic capacity (VO_2 max). However, other factors that influence performance also can guide training goals. These include increasing exercise economy and efficiently using fat as a fuel source, increasing lactate threshold, and increasing the size of Type I muscle fibers. There are several types of aerobic-training programs, and each of these affects one or more training goals. The heart rates associated with the training goals will be presented as a percentage of the MHR and a percentage of the HRR.

Training Goal

Training methods for increasing VO_2 max:

- Interval training uses three to five minutes of running at intensities close to VO_2 max with rest periods (work/rest ratio of 1:1). Running at 85% to 95% of VO_2 max is equivalent to 92% to 98% of MHR or 85% to 95% of HRR.

- Fartlek training combines easy aerobic exercise (~70% VO_2 max) with short bouts of fast exercise (85% to 95% VO_2 max). Heart rate during Fartlek training should be 81% of MHR or 70% of HRR during the easy exercise and between 92% to 98% of MHR or 85% to 95% of HRR during the fast exercise.

Training methods for improving exercise/running economy:

- Pace/tempo training is usually twenty to thirty minutes of running at or slightly above race pace. The intensity should be close to the lactate threshold. In a trained individual, lactate threshold is usually about 80% of VO_2 max, which is equivalent to 88% of MHR or 80% of HHR.

- High-intensity interval training consists of repeated short bouts (thirty to ninety seconds) of high-intensity exercise (at or above 90% VO_2 max) with intermittent periods of short rest. The training heart rate associated with this type of training is 96% to 100% of MHR or 90% to 100% of HRR.

- Fartlek training (aerobic exercise at ~70% VO_2 max and short bouts of fast exercise at 85% to 95% VO_2 max; heart rate 81% of MHR or 70% of HRR and between 92% to 98% of MHR or 85% to 95% of HRR, respectively)

Training methods for increasing the efficient use of fat as a fuel source:

- LSD running requires a running duration of thirty minutes to two hours at a heart rate that is approximately 81% of MRR or 70% HRR (equivalent to 70% of VO_2 max)

- Fartlek training (aerobic exercise at ~70% VO_2 max and short bouts of fast exercise at 85% to 95% VO_2 max; heart rate 81% of MHR or 70% of HRR and between 92% to 98% of MHR or 85% to 95% of HRR, respectively)

Training methods for increasing lactate threshold:

- LSD running to improve the clearance of lactate from the body and ultimately improve lactate threshold (thirty minutes to two hours at approximately 81% of MRR or 70% HRR, equivalent to 70% of VO_2 max)

- Pace/tempo training (twenty to thirty minutes of running at or slightly above race pace, close to the lactate threshold)

- High-intensity interval training (repeated short bouts at or above 90% VO_2 max with intermittent periods of short rest; training heart rate 96% to 100% of MHR or 90% to 100% of HRR)

- Fartlek training (aerobic exercise at ~70% VO_2 max and short bouts of fast exercise at 85% to 95% VO_2 max; heart rate 81% of MHR or 70% of HRR and between 92% to 98% of MHR or 85% to 95% of HRR, respectively)

Training methods for increasing the recruitment of Type I muscle fibers:

- Chronic use of LSD running affects the metabolic characteristics of muscles, causing a shift from Type IIx to Type I muscle fibers.

Outcomes Associated With the Manipulation of Training Volume

Training volume is one variable that can be manipulated in order to progress an exercise-training program. Increasing training volume can result in physiological adaptations to increased physical stress. General adaptation syndrome (GAS) occurs when the body is subjected to external loading. Firstly, the athlete will experience soreness, stiffness, and decreased performance (alarm phase). Secondly, the body will return to normal (resistance phase). Thirdly, the body will adapt and the athlete's muscle mass and strength will increase (supercompensation phase). If training volume is increased and the athlete is unable to adapt, the athlete may experience overload resulting in overtraining syndrome.

Decreasing training volume and intensity – called *tapering* – is a key part of an endurance athlete's preparation for important competitions. A taper may last between seven and twenty-eight days and it allows the athlete's body to completely recover from training and build muscle and liver glycogen storage. The elevation of the athlete's performance capacity resulting from tapering is sometimes referred to as supercompensation. In contrast, if exercise volume and intensity decrease (resulting from illness, injury, etc., the athlete will begin to lose the physiological adaptations achieved from training, which is called *detraining.*

Volume Based on the Training Goal

Muscular Endurance: Resistance programs focused on improving muscular endurance require performing many repetitions (at least 12) per set with lighter loads and completing 2-3 sets.

Hypertrophy: Resistance programs focused on hypertrophy require athletes to use heavier loads and complete fewer repetitions than they would if they were training for muscular endurance. Hypertrophy is defined as developing larger muscles. There are two forms of hypertrophy: sarcoplasmic hypertrophy and myofibrillar hypertrophy. Sarcoplasmic hypertrophy occurs when muscles adjust to high training volumes. In this form of hypertrophy, the inside of the muscle cell (the sarcoplasm) gets bigger through increasing the proteins, fluid, and mitochondria within the sarcoplasm. Myofibrillar hypertrophy occurs when the contractile proteins of the muscle (myosin and actin) are produced more rapidly after strength exercises. As myosin and actin link to form filaments and the number of filaments increase, the muscle is able to generate more force. Greater force production results in increased muscle strength. Sarcoplasmic and myofibrillar hypertrophy occur together, although the proportion of each type of hypertrophy depends on the type of training. Bodybuilders tend to have more sarcoplasmic hypertrophy while weightlifters tend to have more myofibrillar hypertrophy. Since sarcoplasmic hypertrophy cannot occur without myofibrillar hypertrophy, athletes who want to increase muscle size will generally experience an increase in strength. In general, the guidelines for a resistance-training program aimed at increasing hypertrophy include a goal of 6-12 repetitions of each exercise done for 3-6 sets.

Strength: An athlete may choose to pursue a resistance program that focuses on increasing strength without increasing muscle size. For example, a powerlifter may be stronger than a bodybuilder even though the bodybuilder has larger amounts of muscle mass. Research suggests that optimal strength improvements can be achieved by doing two to five sets of six or fewer repetitions (at the corresponding RM load) for core exercises. Assistance exercises may require only one to three sets.

Power: Lower volumes than required for strength are typically used to maximize the performance quality of the resistance exercise to increase power. Fewer repetitions (1-5 over 3-5 sets) and lighter loads are used to decrease volume.

Aerobic Endurance: In running or other modes of endurance exercise (e.g., cycling, swimming), volume is based on distance. When the intensity of the endurance exercise is known, it is possible to calculate the total metabolic cost, which is equivalent to volume load for resistance exercise. The most efficient way to substantially increase running volume is to do LSD training. Volume can be increased by either increasing the duration of the run over time (i.e., start at thirty minutes and build to two hours) or by increasing the number of days per week that LSD running is completed. Generally, it is better to increase the duration of the LSD training than to increase the training sessions per week. LSD training that is done too often can be detrimental to competitive performance and can alter the muscle fiber recruitment patterns that are required during a race. Increasing the number of intervals completed during high-intensity interval training or increasing the duration of Fartlek training runs can also increase training volume.

Work/Rest Periods and Recovery

The length of rest periods between sets and different resistance exercises depends on three variables: the goal of training, the relative load lifted, and the athlete's training condition. Athletes in poor condition need longer rest periods when starting a resistance-training program. Generally, the amount of rest between sets is positively associated with the load (i.e., heavier loads require more rest, lighter loads require less rest).

Different rest period lengths can lead to a variety of physiological changes and should be considered in the context of the athlete's goals. Longer rest periods promote nervous system and muscular system recovery, while shorter rest periods promote cardiovascular conditioning.

Recommended Rest Period Length Per Training Goal

Muscular Endurance: It is recommended that rest periods between workloads are less than 30 seconds. Because muscular endurance training uses light loads and many repetitions, only a short amount of rest is used. Circuit training typically uses rest periods of 30 seconds or less between resistance exercises.

Hypertrophy: It is recommended that rest periods between workloads are between 30-90 seconds. Research suggests that to increase muscle size it is best to use a limited rest period that does not allow the athlete to fully recover before starting the next set. Strength and conditioning professionals should recognize that resistance exercises using large muscle groups might require extra recovery time because of the metabolic demands of the exercises.

Strength: It is recommended that rest periods between workloads are 2-5 minutes. Maximal or near-maximal repetitions require longer rest periods, particularly for lower-body and all-body structural exercises.

Power: It is recommended that rest periods between workloads are 2-5 minutes, which is similar to the rest periods for developing strength. Maximal or near-maximal repetitions (i.e., heavy load) require longer rest periods, particularly for lower-body and all-body structural exercises.

Metabolic Conditioning: The work-to-rest ratios should be based on the specific energy system stressed. For the phosphagen system, ratios of 1:12 to 1:20 are best, fast glycolysis should use 1:3 to 1:5 work-to-rest ratios, fast glycolysis and oxidative drops to 1:3 to 1:4, and oxidative only is optimized with a ratio of 1:1 to 1:3.

Plyometric Exercises: Plyometric exercises involving maximal effort can improve *anaerobic power*, but adequate recovery time is needed for full recovery. The time between sets is based on a work-to-rest ratio that depends on the volume and type of drill. Work-to-rest ratios are often 1:5 to 1:10. Rest periods between repetitions of certain exercises (e.g., depth jumps) may be five to ten seconds.

Recommended Recovery for Various Types of Training

Resistance Exercise: Typically, one to three days of rest is recommended between resistance-training sessions that focus on the same muscle groups.

Plyometrics: Generally, two to four days of recovery is needed between plyometric-training sessions. This specific number of days will depend on the athlete's sport and the sport season. A specific body area should not be trained on consecutive days.

Aerobic Endurance Exercise: At least one rest day, or active rest day, per week is recommended with endurance-training programs.

Training Frequency

Resistance-training frequency is primarily based on the sport season and the athlete's training status. The training goal(s) associated with each sport season and the athlete's training status will influence the number of weekly resistance-training sessions. For example, if hypertrophy is the training goal for the off-season, the athlete will complete between four and six sessions per week. During preseason, the training goal might be strength. Because there is an increase in sport-specific training in preseason, the athlete will have less time for resistance training and the number of sessions per week will be reduced to three to four sessions per week. In-season, one to three sessions per week are recommended and in the postseason period (active rest), the athlete should participate in zero to three sessions per week, depending on the goal and training status of the athlete. The strength and conditioning professional needs to determine the resistance-training goal for each sport season as well as the number of weekly training sessions that will be possible based on the athlete's entire training program. More advanced athletes may be able to handle four to seven sessions per week while novices may only be able to safely handle two to three sessions per week.

Determining and Assigning Exercise Progression

Determining and assigning exercise progression for an aerobic-exercise program requires the manipulation of the following variables:

- Exercise Mode: The specific type of activity the athlete is doing (examples include swimming, running, cycling, resistance exercise, and plyometrics)

- Training Frequency: The number of exercise sessions completed daily or weekly

- Exercise Duration: The length or amount of time of the training session or bout of aerobic exercise

- Training Intensity: The amount of effort expended during a training session

Aerobic-Exercise Progression
Progression starts with increases in the frequency, intensity, and/or duration of aerobic endurance exercise; however, these increases should not be greater than 10% per week. Elite athletes reach a point where it may not be feasible to increase the frequency or duration of exercise, so progression will involve the manipulation of the intensity of the exercise. Exercise intensity should be monitored using RPE, heart rate, or METS (if machines provide this information) depending on which method was originally used to determine the original exercise intensity prescription. At least one recovery day, or active recovery day, should be included each week.

Plyometric-Training Program Length and Progression
Most plyometric-training programs are six to ten weeks in length; however a four-week plyometric program has been shown to improve vertical-jump height. Similar to many of the other plyometric-training variables, there is limited research examining the effectiveness of programs having varying lengths, so the optimal program length has not been determined. It should be noted that doing plyometric training throughout the season can be beneficial for athletes in sports that require quick and powerful movements. Because plyometrics are a type of resistance training, program progression should follow the principles of progressive overload, which systematically increase training intensity, volume, and frequency in varying combinations. The strength and conditioning professional develops the training schedule and progressive overload based on the sport, training phase, and design of the strength and conditioning program. Athlete experience, sport requirements, and sport season are used to determine the length and progression of the plyometric-training program. Remember that plyometric training is added to an athlete's strength and conditioning program in order to develop more power.

Resistance-Training Progression
Timing of Load Increases
Two-for-Two Rule: The two-for-two rule provides a conservative guideline of structure and consistency for determining when an athlete's training load should be increased across training sessions. Using the rule allows athletes to understand how their training load progresses for each exercise and that sustained performance is needed in order for progression to occur. The rule indicates that when an athlete is able to do two additional repetitions during the last set of the exercise and the athlete does this in two consecutive sessions, the weight should be increased at the next training session.

Quantity of Load Increases

Making the decision to increase load can be difficult. The strength and conditioning professional must consider the athlete's physical condition as well as the body area where the load increase will occur. An athlete who is sleep deprived or who has a poor diet will not be able to increase the training load as readily as an athlete who is well rested and eats balanced meals. Also, an athlete who trains too frequently will not be able to progress as quickly as an athlete who gets an appropriate amount of rest between training sessions.

There are general guidelines for increasing load; however, the amount of variation in the exercises and volume loads will significantly affect what load-value increases are appropriate for a specific athlete. Guidelines for specific load increases, as well as relative load increases, can be used to determine load progression. The general recommendations for absolute load increases for weaker, smaller, or less-trained athletes are 2.5 lbs to 5.0 lbs (1 kg to 2 kg) for upper body exercises and increases of 5 lbs to 10+ lbs (2 kg to 4+ kg) for lower body per week. Stronger, larger, or more-trained athletes may increase upper body loads by 5 lbs. to 10+ lbs. (2 kg to 4+ kg) per week and lower body loads by 10 lbs to 15+ lbs (4 kg to 7+ kg) per week. Relative load increases of 2.5% to 10.0% for all athletes can be used rather than absolute load-increase values.

Periodization

Periodization is a training plan that uses logical phases of training, during which training variables are manipulated to produce physiological adaptations, manage fatigue, minimize overtraining, and promote maximum athletic performance. The periodization plan includes all aspects of training that are planned over a specific period of time (typically one year or, in some cases, two to four years). The preplanned training loads, load volumes, and training intensities are designed to apply the training stress necessary to cause adaptive responses in the athlete. Periodized training consists of segments that are organized around the athlete's sport season and sport activities in a way that will allow training adaptations to occur at appropriate times, thereby improving the athlete's competitive performance.

Macrocycle
The macrocycle is the primary periodization component consisting of the entire annual training program. A macrocycle is typically a year but can be several months or, in rare cases, up to a four-year developmental plan (e.g., Olympic training cycle). The macrocycle consists of smaller segments that are used to focus on specific aspects of training in order to develop the specific athletic qualities required for the athlete to peak and perform optimally during competition. A common macrocycle divides the athlete's training year into off-season, preseason, in-season (i.e., competition), and postseason periods.

Mesocycle
A mesocycle is a segment of the macrocycle that is generally a block of two to six weeks (four weeks is the most common length). This time frame has been shown to optimize adaptations to training.

Microcycle
A microcycle is the shortest training segment, lasting from several days to weeks. Variables like intensity and volume can be manipulated to alter the athlete's training within the microcycle segment. The manipulation of the microcycle training is an important part of tapering athletes for competition. An athlete's training progress can be consistently monitored and altered across the microcycle.

Preparatory Period
The preparatory period is usually the starting point of the periodization training plan. It is usually the longest period and most often corresponds to the off-season when there are no competitions. This

period establishes a base level of conditioning that will provide the athlete with the ability to tolerate increased training intensity. The preparatory period is divided into the general preparatory phase and the specific preparatory phase.

General Preparatory Phase
The general preparatory phase takes place during the early part of the preparatory period and focuses on developing the general physical conditioning that will be required for the athlete to handle more intense training. The conditioning during this phase consists of high-volume and low-intensity training and includes activities like slow distance swims, resistance training using high repetitions and light-to-moderate loads, and low-intensity plyometrics.

Hypertrophy/Strength-Endurance Phase
The hypertrophy phase, also known as the strength-endurance phase, takes place during the general preparatory phase. The two primary goals of the hypertrophy phase are to develop the athlete's physical endurance base and increase lean body mass. This phase uses low-to-moderate intensity and high volume. For example, exercises might consist of three to six sets of eight to twenty repetitions at 50% to 75% of 1-RM.

Specific Preparatory Phase
The specific preparatory phase builds on the general conditioning base and begins to focus on more sport-specific training.

Basic Strength Phase
The basic strength phase occurs during the specific preparatory phase and focuses on increasing the strength of primary sport-specific muscle groups. This is achieved by using higher-intensity and moderate-volume training. For example, exercises might consist of two to six sets of two to six repetitions at 80% to 95% of 1-RM.

First Transition Period
The first transition period is the training segment between the preparatory phase and the competitive period. This "precompetitive" period focuses on converting strength into power. The last week of the first transition period focuses on recovery with reduced work volume and intensity, thus allowing the athlete to recover from training in preparation for the competitive period.

Strength/Power Phase
Definitions:

- Strength: The ability to produce force

- Power/Explosive Strength: The time rate of doing work (power = work x time)

- Work: The product of the force exerted on an object, and the distance the object moves in the direction in which the force is exerted (also called displacement; work = force x displacement)

The strength/power phase is the primary phase of the first transition period (the second segment of the preparatory period). The focus during the strength/power phase is on increasing training intensity to pre-competition levels. Resistance-training exercises consist of low-to-very-high loads and low volumes. For example, exercises might consist of two to five sets of two to five repetitions at 30% to 95% of 1-RM.

Competitive Period

The focus of the competitive period (also called the competition period) is preparing the athlete for competition. This is achieved by increasing strength and power. Training intensity increases and volume decreases. Resistance-training exercises consist of moderate and high intensities and moderate volumes. Individual sports with a competition period of several weeks (i.e., fencing or judo) will use a peaking program, while team sports with competition periods of several months will use a maintenance program.

Peaking Programs: The objective of a peaking program is to get the athlete in peak performance condition for one to two weeks. To reduce fatigue, the training progressively shifts from higher-intensity to lower-intensity training as the athlete goes through the taper prior to competition. Resistance-training exercises consist of very high to low intensities and low volumes. For example, exercises might consist of one to three sets of one to two repetitions at 50% to 93% of 1-RM. Trying to extend a peak beyond one to two weeks will decrease fitness and reduce performance capacity.

Maintenance Programs: The extended duration of the competitive period requires training to be manipulated across microcycles. Alterations in training intensity and volume effectively maintain strength and power while simultaneously controlling the fatigue that results from frequent competitions. Resistance-training exercises will be modulated between moderate-to-high intensities and moderate volumes. For example, resistance exercises would consist of approximately two to five sets of three to six repetitions at 85% to 93% of 1-RM. It should be noted that the two-to-five-set recommendation does not include warm-up sets and is the target number of sets for core exercises only.

Second Transition Period

The second transition period (also called active rest or restoration period) is between the competitive period and preparatory period of the next macrocycle and is typically one to four weeks in duration. During this period, intense training is avoided in order to allow athletes to recover from injury and get both physical and mental rest. If this period lasts longer than four weeks, the preparatory phase will need to be longer to allow enough time for the athlete to regain a conditioning base. During this period, athletes can participate in other recreational sports and resistance training, if desired, using very low volumes and loads.

Unloading/Deloading Week

The second transition period can be designed to have one-week rests between three-week training phases. The week of rest allows the body to "unload" in preparation for the upcoming training.

Periodization Models

Linear Periodization Model: This is the "traditional" resistance-training periodization model. It is called linear because of the gradually progressive mesocycle intensity increases, but this is actually a misnomer because the linear model has substantial amounts of variation in intensities and volumes at the microcycle level and across the mesocycle. Resistance-training exercises across days consist of the same number of sets and repetitions, but the load varies across days. This type of training results in volume-load changes.

Undulating Periodization Model: Also called the nonlinear periodization model by individuals in the strength and conditioning industry, the undulating periodization model has daily fluctuations in training intensities and volumes for core resistance-training exercises. During a training week, one day may be focused on strength (four sets with a 6-RM load), the second day might focus on power (five sets with a 3-RM load), and the third set might focus on hypertrophy (three sets with a 10-RM load).

Training Variations Based on a Sport Season

Professional and collegiate sports usually have an annual schedule broken into four sport seasons: off-season, preseason, in-season, and postseason. In periodization, the macrocycle is typically an annual training plan, so the four sport seasons easily relate to the training periods in the periodization model.

<u>Off-Season</u>

Off-season lasts from the end of postseason to the beginning of preseason with the actual duration of the off-season varying greatly depending upon the sport. An athlete in the off-season must build up cardiorespiratory strength gradually with low-intensity and long-duration training before progressing to a shorter and more intense program in the preseason and preparing for competition. The off-season occurs during the preparatory period. The general and specific preparatory phases (subdivisions of the preparatory period) are broken into mesocycles. The mesocycles focus on hypertrophy/strength endurance and basic strength and are planned based on an athlete's needs and preparation for the competition period. For example, if basketball players need to increase muscle mass, they would complete a greater number of mesocycles that focus on the hypertrophy/strength-endurance phase.

<u>Preseason</u>

Preseason follows the completion of the off-season and leads into the first competition. Preseason often coincides with the first transition period and focuses on the strength/power phase with an increase in the intensity of training. Preseason training builds on the physical capacity developed during off-season training with the goal of increasing performance capacity for the competitive period.

<u>In-Season</u>

Also known as the competition period, the in-season consists of all the competitions and tournament games for the year.

<u>Postseason</u>

Postseason corresponds to the second transition period and begins after the final competition. Postseason provides athletes with an active rest period during which intense training is avoided. Because detraining can occur during postseason, longer postseasons require longer preparatory periods during the next year's off-season.

Designing Programs for an Injured Athlete During the Reconditioning Period

<u>Common Injuries</u>
- Dislocation: A joint is completely displaced from its articulating surfaces.

- Subluxation: A joint is partially displaced from its articulating surfaces.

- Strain: A macrotrauma to muscles causes the muscle tissues to partially or completely tear.

- Sprain: A macrotrauma injures joint ligaments.

- Macrotrauma: A tissue (i.e., bone, muscle, ligaments, etc.) is overburdened, which results in poorer tissue health and quality.

- Microtrauma: A tissue becomes overstressed from overtraining.

- Tendinitis: A tendon becomes inflamed from stress on the joint due to overuse or surface resistance.

- Fibrosis: Scar tissue forms near joints. This age-related disorder affects the health and quality of muscle tissue and can limit joint movement, thus increasing the risk of injury.

Tissue Healing and Reconditioning
Inflammatory Response Phase
This phase is characterized by pain, swelling, redness, increases in inflammatory cells, and reduced collagen production; it typically lasts two to six days. Inflammation starts immediately after injury and can occur both locally at the site of injury and systemically.

Treatment Goals: The suggested treatment to minimize inflammation and decrease pain is PRICE (protection, rest, ice, compression, and elevation). Electrical stimulation may also be used as a treatment. Maintenance of the function of the cardiovascular system and the strength, endurance, and power of the musculoskeletal tissues is important.

Exercise Strategies: The injured area should get rest. Exercises that do not directly involve the injured area can be performed after the strength and conditioning professional discusses the exercises that are indicated and contraindicated for the injury with the athletic trainer.

Fibroblastic Repair Phase
This phase is characterized by decreased inflammatory cell activity, collagen-fiber production, and organization. It starts after inflammation materials have been removed and may last up to two months. The breakdown of nonviable tissue (catabolism) due to injury occurs and nonviable tissues are replaced. To increase the integrity of the tissue, scar tissue and capillaries form in the injured area with Type III collagen being produced and put down transversely along the injured structure.

Treatment Goals: The suggested treatment for this phase is to continue reducing inflammation, minimize muscle atrophy, maintain ROM (minimize contractures and adhesion formation), and improve strength and function. Minimizing the joint deterioration and muscle atrophy of the injured area is the primary treatment goal.

Exercise Strategies: Under the consultation of a team doctor or athletic trainer, submaximal isometric exercises can be performed if the athlete is free of pain. Isokinetic exercise with equipment can be used; however, this method is limited because few sport motions occur at a constant speed. Isotonic exercises can be performed with concentric and eccentric muscle movements to increase the strength of the healing tissue. Proprioceptive exercises can be used to improve neuromuscular control. These include completing common exercises such as push-ups on uneven surfaces and using equipment (e.g., mini trampolines, balance boards, or stability balls) that create uneven surfaces for training. Removing visual input by closing the eyes during these exercises can further develop balance. To further challenge the body, the final exercise strategy is to increase the speed of exercises being performed. Note that active-resistance exercises focused on the injured tissue should NOT be performed in order to protect the fragile new tissue.

Maturation-Remodeling Phase
The final phase of tissue repair is characterized by stronger Type I collagen getting laid down longitudinally to increase the strength of the new tissue. Tissue remodeling can continue for more than one year after injury. The realignment and remodeling of the collagen fibers due to increased loading and hypertrophy cause the stressed collagen fibers to realign along the maximally efficient lines of stress, thus allowing the tissue to become more organized and have increased strength.

Treatment Goals: The treatment goals for this phase are to return to the prior level of function, regain full ROM, and go back to the sport activity. Sport-specific exercises can be added in order to apply progressive stress to the injured area.

Exercise Strategies: Functional sport-specific rehabilitation and reconditioning exercises that mimic the demands of the sport should be introduced along with functionally specific strengthening exercises that are consistent with the speed requirements of the sport. Examples of such exercises include closed kinetic chain exercises, joint-angle-specific exercises, more challenging neuromuscular control exercises, and exercises that require velocity-specific muscle activity.

Progression of Rehabilitation and Reconditioning Exercises
Strength and conditioning professionals should use their experience designing programs for uninjured athletes and apply it to the development of reconditioning and rehabilitation programs for injured athletes. The goals of rehabilitation and reconditioning training need to be determined so that a program can be developed that will help the athlete return to the sport as soon as possible.

Resistance-Training Program Design for Rehabilitation and Reconditioning
- DeLorme Program: Uses a pyramid-style design using three sets of ten repetitions that progress from light to heavy loads. For example:

  - Set #1: Ten reps at 50% of ten-repetition max (10-RM)
  - Set #2: Ten reps at 75% of 10-RM
  - Set #3: Ten reps at 100% of 10-RM

- Oxford Program: Very similar to DeLorme's program except the progression of the three sets goes from heavy to light loads. For example:

  - Set #1: Ten reps at 100% of 10-RM
  - Set #2: Ten reps at 75% of 10-RM
  - Set #3: Ten reps at 50% of 10-RM

- Daily Adjustable Progressive Resistive Exercise (DARPE): More manipulation of the intensity and volume of exercises is allowed by the DARPE training system as compared with the DeLorme and Oxford programs. DARPE consists of four sets with a variable number of repetitions. The number of repetitions can range from ten during the first set to one during the fourth set. For example:

  - Set #1: Ten reps at 50% of estimated 1-RM
  - Set #2: Six reps at 75% of estimated 1-RM
  - Set #3: The maximum number of reps that can be completed at 100% or 1-RM
  - Set #4: Performance during the third set determines adjustment to be made to the resistance for the final set.

- Individualizing Resistance Exercise Programs for Injured Athletes: The resistance programs discussed above have been shown to increase muscle strength and might be appropriate to use for some rehabilitation resistance-training programs. The lack of flexibility within these programs makes it difficult to individualize the program to be sport-specific for the injured athletes. Similar to programs for uninjured athletes, programs for injured athletes should follow the specific adaptation to imposed demands (SAID) principle, which says the specific demands placed on a system will cause that system to adapt. Applying the SAID principle to the resistance-training goal requires the design of the resistance program to be based on those exercises that will achieve the training goal.

Instability-Based Exercises for Injury Rehabilitation
Note that instability-based exercises are used in rehabilitation. They have been shown to effectively reduce lower back pain and enhance the stabilization of knee and ankle joints as a result of more efficient soft-tissue stabilization of the joints. Research studies have shown that *anterior cruciate ligament (*ACL) injury risk may be reduced with the use of instability devices, particularly after an ACL injury has been rehabilitated.

Aerobic and Anaerobic Training Program Design for Rehabilitation and Reconditioning
There is no research evidence to support the use of a specific aerobic-training program for rehabilitation. The strength and conditioning professional should develop an aerobic-training program that is sport specific and replicates the metabolic demands required during sport performance. The rehabilitation/reconditioning program design should account for contraindicated exercises based on the injury, but it can be developed based on the prescription guidelines used for healthy athletes. A sport such as wrestling has both aerobic and anaerobic metabolic demands, so interval training is appropriate. Sports with anaerobic metabolic demands – such as powerlifting – need to focus on maintaining anaerobic fitness. Aerobic and anaerobic training can be modified in order to allow injured athletes requiring these types of training to maintain their aerobic and anaerobic capacities. During the inflammatory phase, the injured area should not be stressed. There are many strategies for modifying aerobic and anaerobic training during this phase in order to allow maintenance of aerobic capacities. Alternative forms of aerobic exercise can be utilized. Athletes with injuries to the upper body can use lower-extremity exercises such as cycling and deep-water running, while athletes with lower-body injuries can use upper-body ergometers.

Consider a field-hockey athlete that has an acute injury to the left ankle. Initially during the inflammatory phase, there will be numerous contraindicated exercises for lower-extremity strengthening. However, upper-body resistance and aerobic exercises can be done in order to maintain muscular strength, endurance, and cardiorespiratory fitness. Exercises to strengthen the uninjured lower extremity can also be performed, such as single right-leg squats with weights. The strength and conditioning professional needs to ensure that the injured area is protected, so modifications may need to be made to single-leg exercises.

In another example, the goals of a marathon runner with a patellofemoral injury in the inflammatory response phase will be to maintain cardiorespiratory fitness, muscular strength and endurance in the adjacent joints and muscles, and avoid exercise that requires muscular activity from the quadriceps, as this area must be rested to reduce inflammation. During this phase, cardiovascular exercise that does not exacerbate the pain or increase knee movement is allowable, such as upper body ergometer work. In the fibroblastic repair phase, the athlete may begin using a step machine or stationary bike depending on the decisions of the sports-medicine team, again, as long as it does not exacerbate the knee. Water-based exercises may also be considered. The athlete can perform isometric quadriceps strengthening at full knee extension (progressing to multiple angles) and progress to pain-free isotonic quadriceps strengthening, based on recommendation of the sports-medicine team. With continued progress, the runner should be able to perform two to three sets of fifteen to twenty repetitions of resistance exercises using submaximal intensity ($\leq$50% 1-RM). Finally, in the maturation-remodeling phase, the athlete can start running again, gradually increasing distance and speed. He or she can increase knee ROM as tolerable and add lunges and squats. The intensity of resistance exercises can increase to 50% to 75% of 1-RM (maximal intensity).

Practice Questions

1. Before designing a strength and conditioning program for an athlete, what step should the strength and conditioning professional take to get useful information about the athlete and his or her sport?
   a. Create a long-term plan.
   b. Begin selecting exercises.
   c. Perform a needs analysis.
   d. Determine the athlete's rate of perceived exertion.

2. Which of the following shows the correct dynamic correspondence and training volume?
   a. 120 to 140 repetitions of lower-body plyometrics for a beginner basketball player
   b. 80 to 100 repetitions of upper-body plyometrics for a beginner baseball player
   c. 100 to 120 repetitions of lower-body plyometrics for an advanced volleyball player
   d. 80 to 100 repetitions of upper-body plyometrics for an intermediate soccer player

3. After completing a needs analysis, a strength and conditioning professional determines that an athlete needs improved range of motion for sprinting. Which training method would be best for reaching this goal?
   a. Mobility training
   b. Tactical metabolic training
   c. Pace/tempo training
   d. Repetition training

4. An athlete is performing three sets of chest presses with six repetitions per set. Using the two-for-two rule, how should the athlete increase his or her training load?
   a. By performing eight repetitions on the third set for the next two training sessions
   b. By performing five sets of six repetitions for the next two sessions
   c. By adding two additional training sessions every two weeks
   d. By performing the eccentric and concentric phases of the chest press for two seconds each

5. Which of the following factors would NOT affect an athlete's ability to increase his or her training load?
   a. Lack of sleep
   b. Poor diet
   c. Training too often
   d. Focusing on core exercises

6. Which physiological adaptation is expected after an athlete has participated in an aerobic-training program?
   a. Heart rate reserve decreases and resting-heart rate increases
   b. Heart rate reserve increases and resting-heart rate decreases
   c. Heart rate reserve increases and resting-heart rate increases
   d. Heart rate reserve decreases and resting-heart rate decreases

7. Which of the following statements about rest periods is false?
   a. Longer rest periods promote nervous-system recovery
   b. Longer rest periods promote muscular-system recovery
   c. Longer rest periods promote cardiovascular conditioning
   d. Shorter rest periods promote cardiovascular conditioning

8. Which of the following is the method for organizing the strength and conditioning program and preplanning an athlete's training load and volume to improve his or her physical ability over a certain amount of time?

    a. Training macrocycle

    b. Mesocycle

    c. Preparatory phase

    d. Periodization

9. Which of the following statements about kinetic chain movements is true?

    a. Pull-ups are a closed kinetic chain movement.

    b. Hamstring curls are a closed kinetic chain movement.

    c. Lunges are an open kinetic chain movement.

    d. Leg extensions are a closed kinetic chain movement.

10. What is an example of an appropriate indication for an injured athlete?

    a. A volleyball player with a rotator-cuff injury does shoulder presses.

    b. A basketball player with a sprained knee does leg extensions.

    c. A tennis player with an elbow injury does squats.

    d. A golfer with lower-back pain does back extensions.

11. Which of the following injury-analysis definitions is correct?

    a. A dislocation occurs when a joint is partially displaced from its articulation surface while a subluxation occurs when a joint is completely displaced from its articulation surface.

    b. Macrotrauma to joint ligaments is called a strain, while macrotrauma to muscle tissue is a sprain.

    c. When tissues are overburdened and their health is negatively affected, a macrotrauma occurs and when tissues have been overtrained or have not had time to recover, a microtrauma occurs.

    d. Tendinosis occurs when a tendon becomes acutely inflamed after a joint is overused, experiences excess force, or is overtrained.

12. Arrange the following three steps to reflect to process by which tissue healing occurs:

    I. Tissue repair

    II. Inflammation

    III. Tissue remodeling

    a. I, II, III

    b. II, I, III

    c. II, III, I

    d. III, II, I

13. An athlete wants to increase muscular hypertrophy for a bodybuilding competition. How many repetitions and exercises should be assigned to optimize success in the stated goal?

    a. Six to twelve repetitions per set; three exercises per muscle group

    b. Two to four repetitions per set; three exercises per muscle group

    c. Fifteen repetitions per set; three exercises per muscle group

    d. Six to twelve repetitions per set; one exercise per muscle group

14. Which of the following is true regarding muscle balance?
    a. The strength in opposing muscle groups must be equalized.
    b. The strength ratios in antagonist muscle groups must be improved.
    c. Muscle balance is not an integral part of a strength-training program.
    d. Even if an athlete has improper muscle balance, the body will maintain its normal movement patterns during exercises.

15. Which type of exercises give muscle tissue the most stimulation and are beneficial for limited training time and which type of exercises involve the core muscles and should be the basis of training programs?
    a. Multi-joint; Assistance
    b. Structural; Primary
    c. Primary; Assistance
    d. Multi-joint; Structural

16. An athlete has limited time to train. She wants to improve mental focus and lose body fat. Which type of training would benefit her most?
    a. Split-routine training
    b. 1-RM
    c. Circuit training
    d. Percentage-based training

17. What type of training will help a soccer player to improve his speed and endurance?
    a. Running up hills
    b. Dragging sleds
    c. Wearing a weighted vest
    d. All of the above

18. An athlete would like to improve strength and power for a weightlifting competition. In which order should she complete the following exercises?
    I. Olympic lifts
    II. Back extensions
    III. Bicep curls

    a. I, II, III
    b. II, I, III
    c. III, II, I
    d. II, III, I

19. Which of the following agility-drill classifications is correctly matched with its description?
    a. Serial drills combine continuous and discrete drills and are sport-specific.
    b. Discrete drills are continuous in nature and are useful for developing running and jumping skills.
    c. Continuous drills are helpful for developing specific movement patterns.
    d. Continuous drills can make athletes stronger and more powerful.

20. How can a coach correct a sprinter who "bounces" when she runs?
    a. The coach should help her to practice swinging her arms correctly during short runs.
    b. The coach should her increase her stride rate.
    c. The coach should advise her to keep her head stable with her eyes focused on a specific target.
    d. The coach should advise her to keep her eyes focused on the ground.

21. How many repetitions and sets should be used when training an athlete for muscular endurance?
    a. Six to twelve repetitions for three sets
    b. Six to twelve repetitions for five sets
    c. Twelve to fifteen repetitions for three sets
    d. Two to six repetitions for five sets

22. Which of the following intensity and duration combinations is appropriate for off-season athletes?
    a. Low intensity and short duration
    b. Low intensity and long duration
    c. Moderate intensity and short duration
    d. High intensity and short duration

23. What information should be given to a football player who wants to improve his reaction time?
    a. Reaction time depends on the muscular system, not the nervous system.
    b. Improving reaction time will also improve performance in explosive activities.
    c. He can improve reaction time significantly by being trained to process information at a faster rate.
    d. He can only make small improvements in his reaction time.

24. After doing chest presses, an athlete complains of soreness, stiffness, and lower performance. What advice could a strength and conditioning professional give her?
    a. "You have trained too hard and will not be able to increase your performance beyond this point."
    b. "Keep training as hard as possible and eliminate your recovery time so that your body will experience super-compensation more rapidly."
    c. "You are experiencing the first phase of GAS. If you give your body time to recover, your symptoms will improve and you will eventually become stronger and have more muscle mass."
    d. "You're in the alarm phase of GAS. You should stop your training immediately and see a physician."

25. Which of the following is NOT an appropriate progression method for promoting physiological adaptations in an athlete during the training phase?
    a. Increasing training-load intensities to improve speed
    b. Increasing training density
    c. Increasing training volume
    d. Changing the duration of rest between sets

26. Which of the following approaches should be used to help an athlete recover from previous training sessions and improve neural patterns while promoting supercompensation?
    a. Linear periodization
    b. Unloading/deloading week
    c. Undulating/nonlinear periodization
    d. Rehabilitation

27. Which of the following exercises would help an athlete restore neuromuscular control after an injury?
    a. Doing bodyweight squats on a flat surface
    b. Jumping on a flat surface
    c. Doing push-ups on a flat surface
    d. Jumping on a trampoline

28. Which of the following movement combinations would be most appropriate for a complex-training model?
    a. Bench press at 80% to 90% for two to three reps; plyometric push-ups for three to five reps
    b. Chest press at 50% to 60% for fifteen to twenty reps; bodyweight sit-ups for twenty-five reps
    c. Back squats at 70% for twelve to fifteen reps; maximum-height box jumps for six to eight reps
    d. Leg press at 70% for twelve to fifteen reps; bodyweight calf raises for twenty-five reps

29. Which of the following statements is true about recovery time and training frequency for endurance athletes?
    a. Athletes training at a low intensity need the same number of training sessions but more recovery time than those training at a high intensity.
    b. Athletes training at a high intensity need the same number of training sessions but more recovery time than those training at a low intensity.
    c. Both athletes participating in high-intensity training and those doing low-intensity training need the same amount of recovery time.
    d. Athletes who are doing high-intensity training sessions should get more time to recover and should train less frequently than low-intensity athletes.

30. Interval training for aerobic athletes and anaerobic athletes is similar in which way?
    a. Intervals last the same amount of time for aerobic and anaerobic athletes.
    b. Rest periods last the same amount of time for aerobic and anaerobic athletes.
    c. Both types of athletes are training at higher levels of intensity compared with their VO_2 max.
    d. Both types of athletes use a 2:1 work-to-rest ratio.

31. Which group of athletes would derive the LEAST benefit from Fartlek training?
    a. Powerlifters
    b. Runners
    c. Swimmers
    d. Cyclists

32. What is the most important part of the stretch-shortening cycle response?
    a. Eccentric phase
    b. Concentric phase
    c. Amortization phase
    d. Series elastic component

33. When an athlete performs bicep curls, which of the following is true regarding the phases of the stretch-shortening cycle?
    a. When the athlete raises the weight, the biceps are in the eccentric phase.
    b. The amortization phase is between the eccentric phase and the concentric phase.
    c. When the athlete lowers the weight, the biceps are in the concentric phase.
    d. The athlete is in the amortization phase after he or she begins the bicep curl.

34. What is true about muscle spindles?
    a. They are the most important feature in the stretch-reflex response.
    b. They are the primary baroreceptive structures in the muscle.
    c. They are sensitive to concentric muscle action.
    d. They are the secondary proprioceptive structures in the muscle.

35. In which phase of a sprint is it most important to have excellent mechanics while moving at the highest possible velocity in the shortest time?
    a. Flight phase
    b. Propulsion phase
    c. Recovery phase
    d. Support phase

36. What is the Karvonen method?
    a. When age is used to predict maximum heart rate
    b. When age is used to calculate target heart rate
    c. When resting heart rate is used to predict maximum heart rate
    d. When resting heart rate is used to calculate target heart rate

37. An athlete does one set of five repetitions of shoulder presses with 50 lb. dumbbells. How can a coach calculate how much work he does during the set?
    a. Work equals the amount of weight he lifted.
    b. The coach can divide the weight he lifted by the number of repetitions.
    c. The coach can multiply the weight he lifted by the number of repetitions.
    d. The coach cannot calculate his work with this information.

38. Which of the following statements is true about fibrosis?
    a. Fibrosis may cause some discomfort but will not affect an athlete's mobility.
    b. There is no link between fibrosis and aging.
    c. Since fibrosis is associated with tissue regeneration, this condition has no effect on the overall health of muscle tissue.
    d. Fibrosis can affect an athlete's movement patterns and lead to acute and chronic injuries.

39. What is the difference between the repetition maximum and 1-RM test?
    a. They are the same test.
    b. The repetition maximum test can help identify an athlete's weaknesses when doing multiple repetitions that may not be identified during a single repetition.
    c. The repetition maximum test requires calculating loading parameters for an athlete when he or she is doing multiple repetitions while the 1-RM test does not have this requirement.
    d. The 1-RM test can be used to establish loading parameters for an athlete while the repetition maximum test cannot be used to establish these parameters.

Answer Explanations

1. C: The needs analysis will help to determine the types of movements and physical requirements of an athlete's sport, how much time he or she has to train for the sport, and whether the athlete is a beginner or advanced athlete. Based on this information, appropriate exercises for developing the specific skills that the athlete needs (i.e., dynamic correspondence) and be selected and the appropriate progression can be planned based on how much time he or she can dedicate to training.

2. B: Dynamic correspondence involves choosing an appropriate exercise for an athlete based on his or her sport. For this question, it is important to note that the number of repetitions for plyometric exercises is related to the skill level of the athlete. Beginner athletes should perform 80 to 100 repetitions while intermediate and master athletes should perform 100 to 120 repetitions and 120 to 140 repetitions, respectively. Lower-body plyometric exercises are beneficial for athletes who need to sprint, jump, and make other forceful lower-body movements. Upper-body plyometrics are important for sports that require throwing, catching, tackling, and blocking.

3. A: Mobility training improves flexibility for athletes who have limited range of motion. Tactical metabolic training uses the athlete's sport to create metabolic conditioning drills that mimic the sport's speed and endurance requirements. Pace/tempo training involves training the athlete at the lactate threshold to improve his or her aerobic- and anaerobic-energy systems for the competition. Repetition training requires the athlete to perform several high-intensity sprints for thirty to ninety seconds back-to-back with long rest periods in between.

4. A: The two-for-two rule provides a method for gradually increasing an athlete's strength-training load. Using this method, the athlete should add two repetitions to the last set for two training sessions in a row. Then, the training load can be increased during the following session. In this question, the athlete should add two repetitions to the third set. Therefore, he or she will do eight repetitions instead of six. The athlete should continue this pattern for two training sessions in a row before increasing the load.

5. D: Core exercises can improve an athlete's strength across his or her whole body in addition to specific muscle groups. However, sleep deprivation, lack of nutrition, and overtraining can all reduce an athlete's ability to increase training load. Rest is an important part of strength training and can help an athlete prevent overtraining. Proper nutrition is essential for fueling the workout and providing the building blocks for developing more muscle mass.

6. B: The heart-rate reserve increases and the resting heart rate decreases. Heart-rate reserve is defined as the difference between the maximal heart rate and the resting heart rate. Even though heart rate initially increases during exercise, resting heart rate decreases as a person adapts to aerobic activity. As resting heart rate decreases, the heart rate reserve will increase because the difference between maximal and resting heart rate will increase.

7. C: Longer resting periods improve conditioning. When an athlete needs to improve cardiovascular conditioning, he or she may decrease resting time to bolster aerobic endurance.

8. D: Periodization involves planning and organizing an athlete's entire training program (strength training, range of motion, conditioning, sports drills, etc.) and planning the training loads and volumes to generate physiological changes in a certain amount of time. The training macrocycle represents the developmental goals for the athlete over the entire training program. The mesocycle breaks the macrocycle into two to six-week segments to reach specific training goals. The preparatory phase is the athlete's offseason or preseason period.

9. A: Open kinetic chain exercises allow the loaded limbs to move freely while closed kinetic chain exercises limit this movement. Pull-ups and lunges are closed kinetic chain exercises because the athlete cannot freely move his or her hands or feet when they are planted on the ground. Hamstring curls and leg extensions allow the limbs to swing freely, so these are open kinetic chain exercises.

10. C: Appropriate indications for injuries requires assigning exercises that do not involve the injured area. A tennis player doing squats can build lower-body strength while allowing the elbow to heal.

11. C: Overburdening a tissue results in a macrotrauma while overtraining a muscle leads to a microtrauma. The definitions in answer Choices *A* and *B* have been switched. In answer Choice *D*, a definition for tendin*osis* is given as acute inflammation, which is tendin*itis*. Tendinosis is chronic inflammation of the tendon.

12. B: The tissue-healing process begins with inflammation or swelling and is followed by tissue repair. During tissue repair, damaged tissues are removed while blood vessels and collagen fibers are formed. In the final remodeling phase, new tissues become stronger and more functional.

13. A: Training for muscular hypertrophy requires six to twelve repetitions. Completing more than twelve repetitions improves muscle endurance, while doing fewer than six repetitions improves strength as long as the resistance lifted poses the appropriate challenge at the given repetition level. Using three different exercises per muscle group can significantly increase muscle growth.

14. B: Muscle balance is crucial for any strength-training program because a lack of balance causes the body to have abnormal movement patterns and increases the risk of injury. Creating muscle balance means to improve strength ratios between opposing muscle groups. An example of muscle balance is a 3:4 strength ratio between hamstrings and quadriceps.

15. D: Multi-joint exercises stimulate muscles the most and allow for the greatest amount of loading during resistance training. Primary exercises are core exercises that are sport-specific and involve large muscle groups and multiple joints. Structural exercises are core exercises that load the spine. Assistance exercises engage small muscle groups and single joints.

16. C: Circuit training improves mental focus and requires an athlete to do a variety of exercises (from most intense to least intense) with little rest in between sets. This training program improves cardiorespiratory function and has a high metabolic cost, which leads to increased body-fat loss.

17. D: Running up hills, dragging sleds, and wearing weighted vests will help the athlete to improve speed by increasing the resistance during aerobic training.

18. A: Exercises should be ordered from most to least technical, with power movements first, core exercises second, and single-joint exercises last. Olympic lifts are power movements and require extensive technique, whereas biceps curls require little technique and involve a single joint.

19. A: Serial drills are sport-specific and combine continuous and discrete drills. Continuous drills have no beginning or end and they are helpful for improving running and jumping. Discrete drills help to develop movement patterns and improve an athlete's strength and power.

20. B: Lengthening the sprinter's push-off and stride will reduce vertical bouncing. Answer Choices *A*, *C*, and *D* are corrections for improper arm swinging, premature upright posture, and neck hyperextension, respectively.

21. C: Performing an exercise for at least twelve repetitions will improve muscular endurance, whereas six to twelve repetitions will enhance muscular hypertrophy and fewer than six repetitions will improve muscular strength.

22. B: An athlete in the off-season must build up cardiorespiratory strength gradually with low-intensity and long-duration training before progressing to a shorter and more intense program in the preseason and preparing for the competition.

23. D: Only small improvements can be made to an athlete's reaction time, because reaction time depends on the nervous system and information-processing rates cannot be trained. Reaction time is not related to improvements in explosive activities.

24. C: This athlete's symptoms and history are consistent with GAS. GAS occurs when the body is subjected to external loading. Firstly, the athlete will experience soreness, stiffness, and decreased performance (alarm phase). Secondly, his body will return to normal (resistance phase). Thirdly, his body will adapt and his muscle mass and strength will increase (supercompensation phase).

25. A: Training intensity must be decreased to improve speed. Increasing training volume and changing the duration of rest periods between sets will also promote physical adaptations in the athlete.

26. B: The unloading/deloading week uses lower training volumes and decreases intensity so that the athlete can recover and be prepared for future training sessions. This training week allows the athlete to continue improving neural patterns and promotes supercompensation.

27. D: Doing exercises on an unstable or uneven surface (i.e., doing bodyweight squats or push-ups on a BOSU) helps to improve neuromuscular control by stimulating and challenging the nervous system in new ways, which necessitates adaptation.

28. A: The complex-training model combines heavy resistance training with intense plyometrics to challenge the nervous and musculoskeletal systems. Only answer Choice *A* combines a heavy resistance exercise (80% to 90%) with intense plyometrics.

29. D: The greater the intensity of training, the more recovery time the athlete needs before the next training session. Therefore, athletes training at high intensity should have fewer training sessions per week than athletes training low intensities.

30. C: Interval training involves working at higher levels of intensity compared with one's VO_2 max. Interval lengths and rest periods are very different. Aerobic athletes use a 1:1 work/rest ratio during interval training.

31. A: Fartlek training is an aerobic endurance-training method that combines lower-intensity exercise with brief sprints or other intervals and is most appropriate for runners, swimmers, and cyclists.

32. D: The series elastic components are the hub of activity for eccentric muscle contractions and involves the muscles and tendons. When muscles and tendons stretch, the series elastic components store elastic energy until there is a concentric contraction. The other answer choices are phases of the stretch-shortening cycle.

33. B: The amortization phase is the transition between the eccentric and concentric phases. A muscle shortens in the concentric phase and lengthens in the eccentric phase. When an athlete begins a biceps curl, this is the concentric phase. When he/she lowers the weight, this is the eccentric phase.

34. A: Muscle spindles are essential to the stretch-reflex response because they are the primary proprioceptive structures in the muscle. Muscle spindles respond to eccentric muscle action.

35. C: The recovery phase is key because the sprinter's body is aligned in a way that will enhance speed.

36. D: The Karvonen method allows for the calculation of target heart rate by using resting heart rate.

37. C: Work can be calculated by multiplying the weight by the number of repetitions. Therefore, this athlete's work = 50 lbs. x 5 repetitions.

38. D: Fibrosis is an age-related disorder that causes scar tissue to form near joints. As a result, fibrosis affects muscle health and quality and can restrict joint movement. Restricted joint movement can affect movement patterns and increase the risk of injury.

39. B: Both tests establish loading parameters; however, the repetition-maximum test will determine how well an athlete can perform multiple repetitions of an exercise at a certain load while the 1-RM test only determines how well he or she can complete one repetition. In order to apply the 1-RM test to an athlete's training load at different intensities, the number of repetitions that should be done at a certain load must be calculated. Both tests are important because an injured athlete may perform one repetition easily but struggle to perform the number of repetitions calculated using the 1-RM.

Organization and Administration

Design, Layout, and Organization of the Strength and Conditioning Facility

Designing a feasible strength and conditioning facility from the ground up requires careful forethought and planning, often involving a committee of trained professionals to achieve the necessary physical goals of the facility in an affordable, realistic manner. There are four phases in the design of a new facility, including:

1. *Pre-design phase*: Determining needs, feasibility, and the master plan.

   o *Needs assessment:* Determines what space, equipment, and layout are needed

   o *Feasibility study (SWOT analysis):* Identifies the strengths, weaknesses, opportunities, and threats, to ensure the business will be financially viable and profitable

   o *Master plan:* Includes the building and construction plan and design, and the budget and operational plan

2. *Design phase*: Finalizing the design and blueprint according to city building codes, while focusing on the flow of the facility in terms of equipment, traffic, personnel, etc.

3. *Construction phase*: This phase involves meeting deadlines and avoiding budget overruns, and is based on the master plan. It is often the longest phase. Efforts should be made to meet project deadlines to avoid increases in cost and litigation concerns.

4. *Pre-operation phase*: Finishing the interior design, hiring staff, and planning daily procedures for smooth operation

Modifying an existing facility can be simpler and less expensive in many cases, but still must include many of the same pre-design and planning elements; this can be more challenging because equipment or building construction may already be set in a certain manner that would be difficult or impossible to modify. In either case, strength and conditioning coaches must bring to the committee thoughts and needs regarding flooring; ceiling height (taking into account the platforms of cardio equipment and weight decks, box jumps, and mirror placement so that athletes and coaches can observe form, which in turn can affect window placement); good ventilation and lighting; and ample margins around each piece of equipment. Most manufacturers publish the footprint of equipment for design planning purposes, and planners should bear in mind the need for close proximity to outlets.

Primary Duties and Responsibilities of the Members of the Strength and Conditioning Staff

It is important that all strength and conditioning staff members uphold the facility's goals, mission, and mindset, bringing a high level of professionalism, honesty, trustworthiness, work ethic, and knowledge to their roles. The NSCA requires that strength and conditioning specialists obtain certification. Duties for each position should be detailed in the business and operation plans, as well as required experience and education, expected salary, and schedule. All staff members should maintain CPR/AED certification, and fully understand and rehearse all emergency procedures to reduce the risk of liability issues.

Policies and Procedures Associated with the Operation of the Strength and Conditioning Facility

During the pre-operation phase, policies and procedures regarding facility and equipment cleaning and maintenance, rules, scheduling, and emergency procedures should be planned, assigned to various personnel in certain cases, and written for distribution to employees. To prevent the spread of microbes, mats and exercise surfaces should be wiped down with germicide agents after every use, particularly those that combat the spread of HIV and hepatitis. Floors also require regular cleaning. Non-absorbent surfaces should be mopped, wooden platforms should be monitored for cracks, and regular dusting should remove and prevent grime buildup; these actions will help keep the floor free of obstacles and prevent slips and falls. Regular maintenance should be performed on all equipment in accordance to the manufacturer's recommendations, and cables, pulleys, and bands should be checked for fraying. Facility rules in regard to appropriate attire and footwear, hours, scheduling and canceling policies, payment methods and prices, locker use, etc. should also be formalized. Staff should be trained and rehearsed in all emergency procedures at least quarterly, and procedures should be posted under telephones.

Safe Training Environment within the Strength and Conditioning Facility

Strength coaches are responsible for creating and maintaining a safe training environment within the facility, including safeguarding athletes from risk of injury, illness, and undue emotional distress. By creating safety protocols, keeping the facility clean and organized, and fostering a supportive environment, these risks can be reduced.

Identifying Common Litigation Issues and Reducing or Minimizing the Risk of Liability

Training facilities should create policies and procedures to reduce possible areas of liability, such as handling injury prevention/risk management during training sessions, reviewing emergency procedures, maintaining confidential records, and retaining comprehensive facility and staff liability insurance. Because many aspects of strength training present inherently high injury risk, training staff should make all attempts to keep the training area safe and up to code, keep the floor clear of tripping hazards, closely monitor every session, make certain first aid supplies and AED machines are in close proximity, ensure equipment is routinely serviced and checked, and insist that staff carry liability insurance. *Personal injury liability insurance* protects against libel, slander, and invasion of privacy. *Professional liability insurance* protects against injuries caused by services or negligence. *Commercial liability insurance* covers individuals and the business against incidents and accidents that occur at the facility and must be purchased by trainers who own their own studios. *Negligence* is a failure to perform at the accepted standard (due care), while *gross negligence* is to do so consciously. In addition to carrying the necessary liability insurance, trainers can defend against negligence claims by documenting all services daily and performing at the highest industry standards.

Symptoms Relating to Overuse, Overtraining, and Temperature-Induced Illness

Coaches should be mindful to pace athletes at an appropriate rate and refrain from giving athletes too much too soon, especially regarding competitions and practices outside of the strength training program, which can lead to overtraining and overuse issues. *Overtraining* is a condition that occurs when an individual trains with too much frequency and/or intensity, causing fatigue, greater injury risk, sleep issues, changes in appetite or body weight, lack of motivation, depression or moodiness, and performance decline. Signs of overtraining also include elevated resting heart rate, soreness that does not resolve within a day or two after exercise (as is normal with resistance training), and increased susceptibility to illness. Similarly, *overuse* injuries, such as stress fractures and tendonitis, can occur when the workload is too high and insufficient rest and recovery leads to tissue damage. Strength coaches should also be aware of temperature-induced illness – particularly heat exhaustion and heat stroke – when training athletes outdoors. Signs can include dizziness, nausea, vomiting, clammy skin, confusion, visual disturbances, headache, weakness, and even heart arrhythmias. To prevent such illness, athletes should be encouraged to drink plenty of fluids; wear light, breathable layers of clothing; take frequent breaks in the shade; reduce intensity in hot, humid environments; or modify the workout to indoor settings.

Referring an Athlete to Seek Input from Allied Health Professionals

While athletes may rely heavily on the advice and expertise of strength coaches, strength and conditioning coaches can only educate on topics within their scope, and must refer athletes to appropriate sources for all else. Strength coaches should maintain a list of physicians and allied health professionals—such as physical therapists, nutritionists, and mental health professionals—whom they respect and trust, to provide competent referrals to athletes outside of their scope of practice. When networking with such professionals, strength coaches should be aware that referrals can work both ways, and that through professional, positive relationships with other local clinicians, they may get referrals back for conditioning programs.

Selecting and Administering Tests to Maximize Test Reliability and Validity

Test selection, proper administration adhering to the set protocol, and trained raters influence the reliability and validity of any given test for an athlete. Some tests are only valid for certain populations, such as the 8 Foot Up and Go test of agility in the elderly. All tests are valid only if they are conducted according to the specified protocol, and tests are significantly less reliable if the rater is unfamiliar with test administration, such as a coach performing skinfold measurements without practice at selecting the correct sites and pinching the tissue appropriately.

Tests Based upon the Unique Aspects of a Sport, Sport Position, and Training Status
Selecting the appropriate tests involves considering the physiological energy systems required by the sport compared to the test, movement specificity, and the athlete's experience with training and testing. To choose the most appropriate tests, strength coaches should perform a needs analysis of the sport and position to determine what aspects of fitness are most important (speed, power, strength, agility, etc.) and therefore should be tested. From there, tests should be selected based on their validity for such fitness components as well as the athlete's training status. For example, a VO_2 max running

assessment should be selected rather than a cycle protocol for a distance runner. This choice will prevent local muscle fatigue from the unaccustomed activity, which would reduce overall performance and achievement of a true maximal result. By the same reasoning, a Wingate test of anaerobic power is probably not a good choice for a basketball player who never cycles; the vertical jump test is preferable.

<u>Test Administration Procedures that Use Equipment, Personnel, and Time Efficiently</u>
When testing individual athletes, strength coaches have more flexibility in test selection because equipment usage, personnel to score or observe tests, and time efficiency are less of a concern. Many coaches, however, will need to test entire teams or multiple athletes at one time, so these become factors of consideration. Field tests typically require minimal equipment and occur outside "in the field" such as the Rockport walk test, 1-mile run, or step test, while laboratory tests such as the Wingate test of anaerobic power require equipment. When testing teams or multiple athletes, field tests may be more appropriate because they do not usually require much equipment. In addition, these tests can be conducted more efficiently by having athletes complete them at the same time.

Administering Testing Protocols and Procedures to Ensure Reliable Data Collection

To ensure reliable data collection and scoring, tests should be conducted according to their established protocols and procedures, and in a logical order so that fatigue and testing error do not confound results.

<u>Testing Equipment and Proper Use</u>
To avoid errors in scores based on equipment malfunction or influence, all testing equipment should be assessed for proper function and be calibrated prior to use in testing. For example, prior to using a metabolic cart to measure expired gases, the cart should be calibrated by entering the environmental data (humidity, barometric pressure, temperature) as well as volume of expired air with the 3L calibration syringe. The use of some equipment also requires that certain preparation steps are followed to produce a valid response. For example, bioelectrical impedance machines to measure body fat are very sensitive to body water levels, so athletes should urinate before the test. In addition, prior to the test they cannot eat or drink for at least 30 minutes, exercise for at least 12 hours, drink alcohol for at least 48 hours, or consume caffeine.

<u>Testing Procedures</u>
Many tests have procedures for a warm-up and require proper rest between trials, but for those that do not have a warm-up built into the test, coaches should make sure that athletes have performed a thorough warm-up of the metabolic and physiologic systems that will be used in the test. For example, if performing a 1RM bench press test, athletes should warm up with light cardiovascular exercise to increase blood flow, heart rate, and muscle perfusion, then complete a few sets with increasing weight below max, to prepare the muscles for the test. Tests should also be recorded in a logical order with the most fatiguing assessments last. Studies have found that strength scores are lower after cardiovascular endurance assessments, but not vice versa, so strength tests should be conducted prior to strenuous distance runs or 300-yard shuttle runs. If tests need to be repeated due to some sort of error, it is usually preferable to revisit them on another day so that any accumulated fatigue from the first attempt does not confound the subsequent re-take.

Testing to Assess Physical Characteristics and Evaluate Performance
Some common physical characteristics can be measured as follows:

Height and weight: physician's scale

Body fat:
- Skinfold measurements: Caliper measurements of subcutaneous fat from pinches of skin tissue at specific body sites are plugged into equations to estimate body fat percentage.

- Plethysmography (BOD POD®): A laboratory tool uses air displacement to calculate volume of the body along with weight to determine body fat.

- Bioelectrical impedance: Bioelectrical impedance analysis uses the principle that fat mass and fat free mass have different resistances to electrical current. When the resistances are measured, body fat percentage can be calculated.

- Infrared: Fat mass and fat free mass are assessed via a specialized infrared-light-emitting probe placed against an area of the body.

- Dual-Energy X-ray Absorptiometry (DEXA): This is a machine that measures bone mineral density.

- Circumference measurements: Circumference measurements with measuring tape at specific body sites are plugged into equations to estimate body fat percentage.

Performance parameters can be measured in some of the following selected examples:

- Muscular strength: 1RM bench press for upper body and 1RM leg press for lower body
- Anaerobic capacity or power: Wingate cycle ergometer test, vertical jump test, Margaria-Kalamen stair sprint test, medicine ball throw
- Muscular endurance: Push-up test, curl-up test
- Aerobic endurance: Cooper 12-minute run test, 1.5 mile run test
- Agility: 25-yard shuttle test, zig-zag test, quadrant jump test, hexagon test, box drill
- Speed: Line drills, 300-yard shuttle test, sprint tests like 50m sprint, plate tapping test for upper body speed
- Flexibility: sit-and-reach test

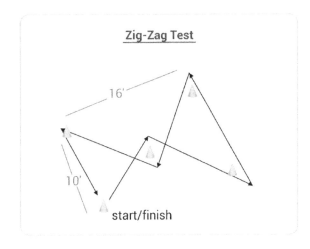

Zig-Zag Test

16'

10'

start/finish

Evaluate and Interpret Test Results

Once tests are completed, the scores are evaluated and the results are translated into usable information to help plan training programs.

Validity of Test Results

Validity refers to the extent to which a test measures what it is intended to measure, such as a strength test actually measuring force production. *Reliability* of a test refers to a test's ability to produce consistent measures. Selecting the appropriate test for an athlete affects the validity and reliability of the test; some tests are valid only for certain populations, and subjective tests become less reliable if they have multiple raters for different administrations of the test.

Typical vs. Atypical Test Results Based on a Sport or Sport Position

Typical assessment scores are somewhat dependent upon sport and position within that sport. For example, highly trained football players tend to have high scores for 1RM bench press and leg press, but score less favorably on cardiorespiratory endurance assessments such as the 1.5 mile run. Most athletes are in sports and positions that suit their physiologic strengths, both through self-selection based on genetic influence as well as years of training to hone certain aspects of fitness. Power athletes tend to have favorable scores for strength and speed assessments compared with endurance athletes, who tend to fair better in muscular and cardiovascular endurance. Dancers, gymnasts, and figure skaters tend to score well in flexibility assessments. Atypical results occur when something other than what should be expected, based on the athlete's training background and genetics, occurs. Atypical results can sometimes indicate that the testing was not conducted correctly or that the athlete failed to perform up to potential for one reason or another in that assessment.

Design of a Training Program Based on Test Results

Each of the recommended fitness assessments has standards that the strength coach can compare an athlete's results to. *Norm-referenced standards,* such as VO$_2$ max score, compare the athlete's performance against that of similar individuals and scores are presented in percentiles. The 50th percentile indicates the athlete performed better than half of the comparative population and worse than half. It is important that the coach reports not just the percentile score, but educates athletes on their scores' relative value. *Criterion-referenced standards* are based on research- and normative-based achievement levels of health and fitness that, if reached, predict lower disease risk for the athlete. These may be lower standards than those likely achieved by athletic populations. Coaches can use the testing results to help in training program planning. Taken together with an understanding of the most important fitness components for a given athlete based on sport and position, coaches can look at the norm-referenced standards for each test score for an athlete to identify the greatest areas of deficit and be sure to emphasize them, along with those that are most important for the position, in training programs. For example, if a baseball pitcher scores in the 90th percentile for upper body 1RM strength, but in only the 70th percentile for muscular endurance based on the push-up test, coaches would want to focus on increasing muscular endurance, both because the athlete is less proficient with endurance (according to percentile rank), but more important, because pitching an entire game requires a high level of upper body muscular endurance.

Practice Questions

1. A marathon runner scores in the 40th percentile for 1RM bench press and the 70th percentile for VO_2 max, based on a 1.5-mile run. Which of the following should a coach emphasize in a training program?
   a. Upper body strength
   b. Cardiovascular endurance
   c. Lower body strength
   d. Upper body endurance

2. Which of the following anaerobic power tests is likely the LEAST optimal choice for a volleyball player?
   a. Vertical jump test
   b. Wingate test
   c. Margaria-Kalamen stair sprint test
   d. Medicine ball throw

3. A tennis player scores in the 60th percentile for 1RM leg press and the 70th percentile on the push-up test. Which of the following should a coach focus more on in a training program?
   a. Upper body strength
   b. Cardiovascular endurance
   c. Lower body strength
   d. Upper body endurance

4. When selecting the most appropriate assessments for an athlete, the strength and conditioning coach should consider which of the following?
   I. The athlete's strengths and weaknesses
   II. The athlete's sport
   III. The athlete's position
   IV. The athlete's training level

   a. All of the above
   b. II, III, IV
   c. I, II, III
   d. II, III

5. Which of the following is true of testing equipment?
   a. It is needed for field-based tests.
   b. It needs to be calibrated prior to use.
   c. It produces more accurate results than tests with minimal equipment.
   d. It makes it easier to test multiple athletes at one time.

6. Prior to a 1RM bench press, an athlete should do which of the following?
   I. A 5 to 10-minute jog
   II. One minute of push-ups
   III. A few sets of submaximal bench presses
   IV. A 300-yard shuttle test

   a. All of the above
   b. I, III, IV
   c. I, II, III
   d. I, III

7. Which of the following does NOT typically affect the validity of an assessment?
   a. Population tested
   b. Order of tests conducted
   c. Test selection
   d. Rater's skill level

8. Which of the following does NOT take place in the pre-design phase of building?
   a. SWOT analysis
   b. Feasibility study
   c. Needs assessment
   d. Finalizing the blueprint

9. How often should emergency procedures be reviewed and rehearsed?
   a. At least every month
   b. At least every week
   c. At least every three months
   d. At least twice per year

10. Which type of insurance protects against claims of libel, slander, and invasion of privacy?
    a. Personal injury liability
    b. Professional liability
    c. Commercial liability
    d. Negligence liability

11. To control the spread of germs in the facility, what should athletes be taught and instructed to do?
    a. Supplement with Vitamin C and zinc
    b. Wear appropriately supportive sneakers
    c. Wipe down all used equipment after use with antibacterial agents
    d. Engage the emergency stop buttons on cardio equipment

12. Which of the following is the correct order of phases for designing a new fitness facility?
    a. Pre-design, design, construction, pre-operation
    b. Design, pre-construction, construction, pre-operation
    c. Pre-design, design, pre-construction, pre-operation
    d. Pre-planning, design, pre-construction, construction

13. What type of score is VO_2 max?
    a. Norm-referenced score
    b. Criterion-referenced score
    c. Reliability-referenced score
    d. Validity-referenced score

14. An elite cross country skier gets a VO_2 max score that indicates she is in the 30th percentile for her age. Which of the following may be true of this performance?
    a. This indicates she has good cardiovascular endurance, which makes sense because of her sport.
    b. This is an atypical result, and there may have been an error in the protocol, equipment, or scoring.
    c. This is an atypical result, and the test should be conducted again after a 5 to 10-minute break.
    d. This makes sense because she is a cross country skier, so her cardiovascular endurance would be low.

15. Which of the following agility tests would NOT be appropriate for a collegiate hockey player?
    a. Hexagon test
    b. 8 Foot Up and Go test
    c. Zig-zag test
    d. Box drills

16. What should strength coaches conduct prior to selecting tests for athletes?
    a. Feasibility study
    b. Needs analysis
    c. SWOT analysis
    d. Body composition assessments

17. In which of the following situations is it necessary to refer to an allied health professional?
    a. An athlete who has questions about pre-workout hydration
    b. An athlete who has performance anxiety but is not ready to address it
    c. An athlete who wants a nutritional plan to add muscle mass
    d. An athlete who has tight hamstrings after increasing training volume

18. Which of the following would best improve time efficiency when testing a large group of athletes?
    a. Conducting field tests
    b. Conducting laboratory tests
    c. Tests that use one piece of equipment, such as a treadmill
    d. Testing athletes one at a time in a particular order

19. Which of the following tests results would be LEAST important for a shot-putter?
    a. 1RM bench press
    b. Push-up test
    c. Box drill
    d. Vertical jump test

20. When a certified strength and conditioning coach fails to perform what is typically considered to be a standard practice of care, it may be deemed to be which of the following?
    a. Negligence
    b. Malpractice
    c. Liability
    d. Scope of practice

21. Which is NOT a symptom of overtraining?
    a. Lowered resting heart rate
    b. Depression or moodiness
    c. Sleep disturbances
    d. Changes in appetite or body weight

22. Which of the following is NOT recommended for an athlete suffering from a heat-related illness?
    a. Move to the shade
    b. Drink fluids
    c. Remove excess clothing
    d. Continue the workout indoors

23. Which of the following is NOT an overuse injury?
    a. Shin splints
    b. Tennis elbow (lateral epicondylitis)
    c. Metatarsal stress fracture
    d. Groin strain

24. What must all strength and conditioning coaches do?
    a. Obtain first aid certification
    b. Be certified strength coaches
    c. Be former competitive athletes
    d. Establish the mission and values for the facility

25. What pieces of equipment should be evaluated prior to every single use?
    I. Medicine balls
    II. Exercise bands
    III. Cables on weight machines
    IV. Emergency stop buttons on cardio equipment

    a. All of the above
    b. I, III, IV
    c. II, III, IV
    d. III, IV

26. In which order would a strength coach recommend administering the following assessments?
    a. Skinfold, push-up test, step test, 1RM bench press, sit-and-reach
    b. Skinfold, step test, push-up test, 1RM bench press, sit-and-reach
    c. Skinfold, sit-and-reach, step test, 1RM bench press, push-up test
    d. Skinfold, sit-and-reach, 1RM bench press, push-up test, step test

27. Which of the following tests results is least important for a soccer midfielder?
    a. 1RM bench press
    b. Cooper 12-minute run test
    c. Box drill
    d. Vertical jump test

28. In designing the interior layout of a training facility, which of the following need to be considered?
    I. Outlet placement
    II. Footprint of machines and equipment
    III. Ceiling height
    IV. Mirror placement

    a. All of the above
    b. I, II, III
    c. I, II, IV
    d. II, III, IV

29. Which of the following tests results is LEAST important for a baseball pitcher?
    a. 1RM bench press
    b. Push-up test
    c. Quadrant jump test
    d. Vertical jump test

30. Body fat assessments include all EXCEPT which of the following?
    a. Skinfold measurements
    b. DEXA scans
    c. BMI
    d. Bioelectrical impedance

31. Practices that strength coaches can implement to foster a safe training environment include all EXCEPT which of the following?
    a. Clearing loose equipment from the floor
    b. Encouraging teamwork and positive, supportive attitudes
    c. Mopping wooden floors and checking wooden platforms for cracks
    d. Keeping weight benches and lifting platforms as close together as possible

32. How can the following image be described?

 a. High reliability, low validity
 b. High validity, low reliability
 c. High reliability, high validity
 d. Low reliability, low validity

33. Which of the following is a field-based body fat assessment?
 a. Skinfold measurements
 b. DEXA scans
 c. BMI
 d. Plethysmography

Answer Explanations

1. B: A marathon runner requires a great deal of cardiovascular endurance. Even though this runner's score was relatively low for 1RM bench press (40th percentile vs. 70th), it is still more important to increase the runner's cardiovascular endurance, given the demands of the sport, compared to upper body strength. The 70th percentile leaves a large margin for improvement. Even though VO₂ max does have a large genetic component, it is likely that this runner can significantly improve marathon times by targeted endurance training. The need for upper body strength is much less important in distance running, although muscular endurance is important.

2. B: The Wingate test is conducted on a cycle ergometer, and so it is least applicable to a volleyball player because that position does not involve biking. Vertical jump, Margaria-Kalamen stair sprint, and medicine ball throws would all be good assessments for this athlete.

3. D: A tennis player relies heavily on upper body endurance (which is measured by the push-up test), so this should be prioritized. Lower body strength is important, but significantly less so, and as this athlete's percentile scores are fairly close and both are within acceptable range, upper body endurance should be more of the focus in training.

4. A: There are many factors that the strength and conditioning coach must consider when selecting the most appropriate assessments for an athlete. There are a wide variety of assessments available for coaches to choose from, and the most appropriate choice should be made by taking into account the athlete's strengths and weaknesses as well as the athlete's sport, position, and training level. Coaches may need to make compromises on some of these variables if the entire team needs to be tested at one time, if tests are only conducted in the field so limited equipment is available, and if there is a tight testing schedule, all of which would not allow for certain test protocols.

5. B: All testing equipment should be assessed for proper function and calibrated prior to use in testing, to avoid errors in scores based on equipment malfunction or influence. For example, prior to using a metabolic cart to measure expired gases, the cart should be calibrated by entering the environmental data (humidity, barometric pressure, temperature) as well as volume of expired air with the 3L calibration syringe. Testing equipment is used in a laboratory, not field-based tests, and it is harder to test multiple athletes at one time because of the need to use the equipment (for instance, a handful of athletes should not be on one treadmill all at once).

6. D: Prior to a 1RM bench press, an athlete should perform a thorough warm-up of the metabolic and physiologic systems that will be used in the test. In this instance, athletes should warm up with light cardiovascular exercise to increase blood flow, heart rate, and muscle perfusion, then complete a few sets with increasing weight below max, to prepare the muscles for the test. The one minute of push-ups is a muscular endurance test and uses the same muscles as the 1RM bench press, which can lead to fatigue before the test. The 300-yard shuttle runs are also fatiguing and have been shown to reduce strength performance, so push-ups for endurance and the 300-yard shuttle should be avoided prior to a 1RM bench press.

7. D: Rater's skill level typically affects the reliability or consistency of a test score. Validity refers to a test measuring what it is intended to measure—such as a strength test actually measuring force production. Reliability of a test refers to its ability to produce consistent measures. Selecting the appropriate test for an athlete affects the validity of a test; some tests are valid only for certain populations. Oher tests are valid only for certain measures (for instance, a 1RM bench press measures upper body strength but should not be used as a measure of upper body endurance). The test order matters in that fatiguing tests should not be conducted prior to less fatiguing tests, or they can confound the results.

8. D: The pre-design phase includes a needs assessment, determining what space, equipment, and layout are needed; a feasibility study or SWOT analysis, identifying the strengths, weaknesses, opportunities, and threats to ensure the business will be financially viable and profitable; and a master plan, including the building and construction plan and design, and the budget and operational plan. Finalizing the blueprint takes place in the design stage.

9. C: Emergency procedures should be reviewed and rehearsed at least quarterly.

10. A: Personal injury liability insurance protects against libel, slander, and invasion of privacy. Professional liability insurance protects against injuries caused by services or negligence. Commercial liability insurance covers individuals and the business against incident and accidents that occur at the facility and must be purchased by trainers who own their own studios.

11. C: To control the spread of germs in the facility, athletes should be taught and instructed to wipe down all used equipment after use with antibacterial agents. The other options are practices that athletes should be taught as well, but that do not help prevent the spread of germs.

12. A: The order of phases for designing a new fitness facility are: pre-design, design, construction, pre-operation.

13. A: VO_2 max is a norm-referenced score. Norm-referenced standards compare the athlete's performance against that of other similar athletes and scores are presented in percentiles. The 50th percentile indicates the athlete performed better than half of the comparative population and worse than half. It is important that the coach reports not just the percentile score, but educates an athlete on his or her score's relative value. Criterion-referenced standards are based on research- and normative-based achievement levels of health and fitness that, if reached, predict lower disease risk for the athlete. These may be lower standards than those likely achieved by athletic populations.

14. B: Cross country skiing requires a high degree of cardiovascular endurance, so the 30th percentile is an atypical score for an elite athlete. There was likely an error in the protocol, equipment, or scoring. The test should not be conducted again after just a 5 to 10-minute break because the athlete will not have recovered from a maximal effort; a re-test should occur on another day.

15. B: The 8 Foot Up and Go test is an agility test for senior citizens, while the others are for healthy, athletic populations.

16. B: To choose the most appropriate tests, strength coaches should perform a needs analysis of the sport and position to determine what aspects of fitness are most important (speed, power, strength, agility, etc.) and should be tested. Body composition assessments are part of the battery of test options, so it would not make sense to perform them prior to testing, as they are part of testing. Feasibility studies and SWOT analysis are part of business planning.

17. C: While coaches are able to provide information and advice pertaining to fitness and training, the scope of practice is limited to these areas and nutrition planning cannot be provided legally by a strength and conditioning professional. Referring the athlete to a registered dietician or nutritionist would be the proper course of action for nutrition planning.

18. A: Field tests typically require minimal equipment and occur outside "in the field," such as the Rockport walk test, 1-mile run, or step test, while laboratory tests such as the Wingate test of anaerobic power require equipment. When testing teams or multiple athletes, field tests may be more appropriate because they do not usually require much equipment. In addition, the tests can be conducted more efficiently by having many athletes complete them simultaneously.

19. C: The box drill test is not the best choice because agility is less important for shot-putters. Shot-putters do need good upper body muscular strength and endurance, as well as some amount of leg power to give momentum to throws, so the 1RM bench press, push-up test, and vertical jump test are appropriate.

20. A: When a certified strength and conditioning coach fails to perform what is typically considered to be a standard practice of care, it may be deemed to be negligence.

21. A: Overtraining is a condition that occurs when an individual trains with too much frequency and/or intensity, causing fatigue, greater injury risk, sleep issues, changes in appetite or body weight, lack of motivation, depression or moodiness, and performance decline. Signs of overtraining also include elevated resting heart rate, soreness that does not resolve within a day or two after exercise (as is normal with resistance training), and increased susceptibility to illness.

22. D: To resolve heat-related illness, athletes should drink plenty of fluids, remove excess layers of clothing, and move to the shade. Once symptoms have set in, it is too late to continue the workout inside. Exercise will need to stop. To prevent heat-illness in the first place, the workout can take place inside.

23. D: Groin strains are typically an acute injury. Overuse injuries such as stress fractures and tendonitis can occur when the workload is too high and insufficient rest and recovery leads to tissue damage.

24. B: All strength and conditioning coaches must be certified strength and conditioning coaches and have CPR/AED certification. First aid is recommended, although not required. The mission and values for a facility may be created by the strength coach, with or without others in the business, but are often created by the owner or manager of the business, prior to hiring a strength coach.

25. C: While medicine balls should be checked weekly or so for cracks, which can cause sand to leak out, unless they are old or get substantial use, they likely are not something that needs to be checked prior to every use. More important, even if they do have sand leaks, they should not injure an athlete when they are starting to fall apart. Exercise bands routinely thin and then can snap and cables fray, both which can be very dangerous. Emergency stop buttons on cardio equipment should also be checked prior to usage.

26. D: NSCA guidelines suggest this order, with #1 and #2 being interchangeable:

1. Skinfold
2. Sit-and-reach
3. 1RM Bench Press
4. Push-up Test
5. Step Test

The reason there are guidelines for the order of assessments is to ensure that one assessment does not affect another. Stretches and measurements of physical attributes should be first since they don't cause fatigue. Agility tests come next, though there were none listed in this practice questions. Muscular strength tests should follow, to optimize peak strength before prematurely fatiguing muscles through drawn out muscular endurance tests like the push-up test. In this case, the muscular test is the 1RM Bench Press. While there should be a rest period following this assessment, note that since it's just "One Rep Max", it won't be too tiring nor will it be aerobic. Next comes sprint tests (none here), and then local muscular endurance tests. Push-ups are a principle example of this. Finally, anaerobic tests and then aerobic capacity tests should be conducted. Steps tests are one of the latter.

27. A: Soccer midfielders need cardiovascular endurance, agility, and lower body power and speed, so the Cooper 12-minute run test, box drill, and vertical jump test are good choices. Upper body strength is less important in this position, so a 1RM bench press is less important.

28. A: The outlet position, equipment footprint, ceiling height, and mirror placement must all be taken into consideration in order to provide athletes and coaches with a safe environment conducive to training of all formats.

29. C: Agility is less important for baseball pitchers, so the quadrant jump test is not the best choice. Pitchers do need good upper body muscular strength and endurance, as well as some amount of leg power to give momentum to pitches, so the 1RM bench press, push-up test, and vertical jump test are more appropriate.

30. C: BMI is a measure of weight relative to height and not body fat. Skinfolds, DEXA scans, and bioelectrical impedance are common assessments for body fat.

31. D: Practices that strength coaches can implement to foster a safe training environment include clearing loose equipment from the floor, mopping wooden floors, and checking wooden platforms for cracks. Emotional safety is enhanced through encouraging teamwork and positive, supportive attitudes. Weight benches and platforms should not be as close as possible; they require a minimum of 36 inches of clearance for walking around them safely, keeping distance between athletes lifting weights, spotting, and preventing injuring a nearby athlete.

32. A: This image shows high reliability because the arrows are consistently in the same area, but low validity because they are not near the bullseye.

33. A: Skinfold measurements are easily conducted on the field with a pair of calipers. With experience, the coach can conduct 7-site or 3-site skinfold measurements on individual athletes in just a few minutes, making it an efficient measurement, even for a large team. BMI does not measure body fat, but rather weight relative to height. DEXA scans and plethysmography are common assessments for body fat, but they take place in medical facilities and not in the field.

Dear CSCS Test Taker,

We would like to start by thanking you for purchasing this study guide for your CSCS exam. We hope that we exceeded your expectations.

Our goal in creating this study guide was to cover all of the topics that you will see on the test. We also strove to make our practice questions as similar as possible to what you will encounter on test day. With that being said, if you found something that you feel was not up to your standards, please send us an email and let us know.

We would also like to let you know about other books in our catalog that may interest you.

ACSM

This can be found on Amazon: amazon.com/dp/1628454903

ACE

amazon.com/dp/1628455411

NASM

amazon.com/dp/1628454296

We have study guides in a wide variety of fields. If the one you are looking for isn't listed above, then try searching for it on Amazon or send us an email.

Thanks Again and Happy Testing!
Product Development Team
info@studyguideteam.com

Interested in buying more than 10 copies of our product? Contact us about bulk discounts:

bulkorders@studyguideteam.com

FREE Test Taking Tips DVD Offer

To help us better serve you, we have developed a Test Taking Tips DVD that we would like to give you for FREE. **This DVD covers world-class test taking tips that you can use to be even more successful when you are taking your test.**

All that we ask is that you email us your feedback about your study guide. Please let us know what you thought about it – whether that is good, bad or indifferent.

To get your **FREE Test Taking Tips DVD**, email freedvd@studyguideteam.com with "FREE DVD" in the subject line and the following information in the body of the email:

> a. The title of your study guide.

> b. Your product rating on a scale of 1-5, with 5 being the highest rating.

> c. Your feedback about the study guide. What did you think of it?

> d. Your full name and shipping address to send your free DVD.

If you have any questions or concerns, please don't hesitate to contact us at freedvd@studyguideteam.com.

Thanks again!

Made in the USA
Columbia, SC
12 May 2019